How to Be a
TEEN
Fashionista

How to Be a
TEEN
Fashionista

Put Together the *Hottest Outfits* and *Accessories* — On Any Budget

CHASE KOOPERSMITH

FAIR WINDS
PRESS
GLOUCESTER, MASSACHUSETTS

FAIR WINDS

Text © 2005 by Chase Koopersmith
Photographs © 2005 by Allan Penn

First published in the USA in 2005 by
Fair Winds Press
33 Commercial Street
Gloucester, MA 01930

09 08 07 06 05   1 2 3 4 5
ISBN 1-59233-162-9
Library of Congress Cataloging-in-Publication Data available

Cover design by Laura Herrmann Couallier
Book design by Peter King and Company
Styling by Chase Koopersmith
Cover makeup by Bonni Flowers
Models' makeup by Bonni Flowers and Francie Paull
Hair by Lawerance Davis and Samantha Thompson
Chase's haircut and color by Martina Harrer
Eyebrows by Janette Cassandra, Cassandra the Wax of the Millennium
Makeup provided by MAC Cosmetics
Cover clothing by Rocawear

Printed and bound in USA

DEDICATION

I dedicate this book, first, to God, because without Him I wouldn't have had the strength to go through the process. He has blessed me by surrounding me with so many beautiful and talented people. I would also like to dedicate this book to my mom, Linda Koopersmith, for her love, support, and everything else she does for me, and to my grandmother, Betty Koopersmith, for believing in me and encouraging me to follow my dreams. Last, but not least, to my friends: Thank you for being there with me through thick and thin. I love you all so much!

Contents

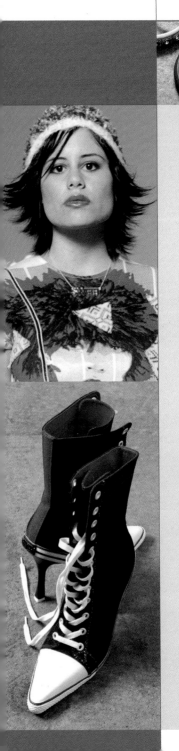

Part One : From Clueless to Best Dressed

Part Two : How to Put an Outfit Together

Part Three : Where to Find It

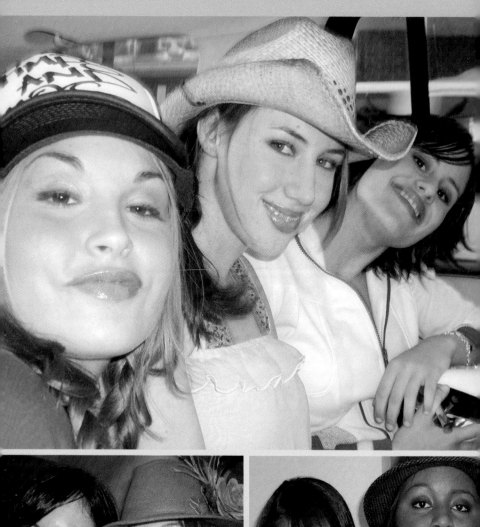

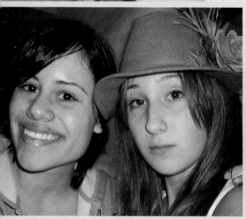

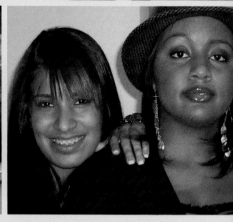

Introduction
How You Can Be a Teen Fashionista

How to Be a Teen Fashionista, Put Together the Hottest Outfits and Accessories—on Any Budget is a how-to book that will increase your ability to put outfits together and help you create more ensembles out of your existing wardrobe. This book came about because many people over the years have asked me how I put my outfits together. It includes tips and places to shop, as well as what looks flattering versus unflattering on your figure. Think of this as an art book helping you create unique masterpieces of your own. Maybe it really isn't considered "art," but creating outfits every day is a way for me to express myself, and I consider that art.

I am a normal teenage girl just like you. I've had my share of trials and tribulations with fashion. I have those days when I don't feel I look my best. Everybody has those low self-esteem days; that's just part of life! However, creating fabulous fashions might just boost your spirits a wee bit so all of a sudden, the day isn't too horrible anymore.

There are always those times when you think you have nothing to wear in your closet. I want to be here and help you through those rough times until you get a chance to get some scissors in your hands to repurpose something, or you get an allowance so you can hit the mall. When your imagination is exhausted, I would like you to pick up this book and be inspired to come up with an amazing ensemble.

My Fashion Evolution

I would like you to join me as I go through my fashion history. I haven't lived all that long, but I wasn't just born with the knowledge of how to coordinate clothing.

It all started after diapers. I was simply the dress queen. My closet contained only dresses, dresses, and more dresses. I was a very stubborn child, and pants just didn't suit me. One experience stands out most in my mind. I was cast in a commercial, and the wardrobe woman told me the dreaded news: I had to wear pants! What would any dress queen do? When I found out that not only was I going to be stuck in some contraption of fabric given the name "pants," but also that the other little girl got to wear a dress, I threw a fit! I must have been a nightmare for my mom. That has to be my fondest memory of being the queen of dresses. Shortly after that, I decided that pants weren't that bad, and I would give them a go.

When I was old enough to dress myself, I chose to wear the same outfit every day. Sure enough, every night my mom would have to wash the "it" outfit. I remember my mom explaining to me that someone was going to ask me why I always wore the same exact outfit. As my mom predicted, my third grade teacher asked if "anything was wrong" in our household. My mom told her the predicament of how I liked to wear only that certain outfit, although I had a closet full of clothes.

To this day, my mom still calls it "the uniform." Looking back on it, it was kind of vintage me, but at the time that was not my intention.

Once I was over the same-outfit-every-day-stage, I began a new style for myself. I decided it was best for me to wear very plain clothing. That included nothing that most little girls my age would wear. I wouldn't wear the fashions that appeared in Limited Too or GapKids. For me, it was all about very simple articles of clothing—that meant no frills, no designs, and definitely no rhinestones or sequins. I still wear simple tanks, sweats, and T-shirts, but that's only when I don't feel like getting dressed up. I don't think I would ever resort to a complete wardrobe of simple clothing now, because, frankly, I love detailed apparel.

In the fifth and sixth grades, it was all about monkey shirts and baggy pants. I guess I wanted to be a skater chick or something, although I didn't know how to skateboard, and still don't. My motto was "Anything with a monkey on it, I'll buy!" I was compulsive when it came to monkeys. I had calendars, pillows, stuffed animals, night-lights, and clothing all decked out in monkey décor. You name it, I probably had it with a monkey on it somewhere. In retrospect, I would consider that my style involved too much monkey business.

I'd have to say that it wasn't until seventh grade that I really transformed from monkey-lover to fashionista. I became more interested in fashion, and I tried to learn more about it whenever I had the chance. I remember that my art teacher, Ms. Cohen, took our class to Otis in downtown Los Angeles. It was then that I decided that I definitely wanted to have a career in the fashion industry when I was grown up.

In the past four years, my individual style hasn't changed much. It has been altered here and there with the passing trends, but for the most part I've been able to cultivate a style I can claim as all my own. Last year, though, I thought it was genius to wear stilettos every day to school. Ladies, this is not a good idea! I am telling you this as a concerned friend. Your feet will never be the same. Wear heels sometimes because they're pretty, but not all the time. In the long run, you will thank me.

Let's Go, Girls!

With a fresh eye, scissors, crystals, and a bit of dough, you too will be able to turn your wardrobe around and become the next teen fashionista! I would like to share my secrets with you. So now it's time to stop reading this introduction and turn the page to the real goodies!

xoxo,

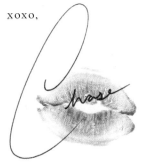

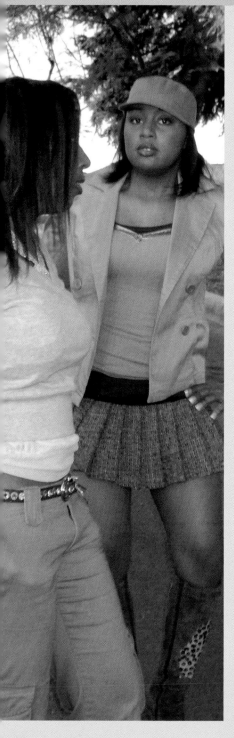

Part One : From Clueless to Best Dressed

1. Your Pluses and Minuses: How to Make the Most of Them

Being the wrestling manager at my school, I witness first-hand what it's like for the wrestlers to make their weight classes. The wrestlers will do practically anything to "make weight," like going all day without food or drink (matches usually start at 3 P.M.), throwing up, and sprinting in jeans and multiple sweatshirts. I realized how utterly grotesque this is, and that at any weight, people are beautiful.

I know that being a teenage girl in high school isn't exactly the easiest thing, and there are so many pressures. One of the pressures that most of my friends and I are faced with is to be thin. It doesn't help when we look at magazines and see these girls nearly our age who have amazing bodies. That is why some girls become obsessed with being thin at any cost. In some cases, they are even worse than the wrestlers.

You shouldn't worry about meeting the "weight class" that you want to be in, because the bottom line is that a few pounds aren't really going to change who you are. So no matter how much you weigh, or how little you weigh, you are gorgeous and should respect your body like you would a temple.

Body Shapes

Determining what you should or should not wear comes down to your body shape. Different styles of clothing can enhance, distract, complement, or exaggerate your pluses or minuses. Start out by defining what body shape you have.

ARE YOU PEAR-SHAPED?

If you're pear-shaped, a look in the mirror will confirm that your bottom half is larger than your top, making you look like a pear. That usually means you don't have as much in the bra department as you'd like, but remember, you make up for that with a bootylicious bottom!

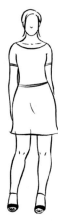

THE PEAR-SHAPED FIGURE

Pluses and minuses

Pear-shaped girls' pluses: You have a big butt, and that is definitely a good thing. Pear-shaped girls' minuses: Your shoulders look small by comparison to your lower half. Here are some tips that will balance your proportions.

What to do

· Coats, jackets, and blazers are good pieces for pear-shaped girls to start with in their wardrobes. Shoulder pads are good, too, but I'm not talking about gigantic chunky ones straight from the '80s. The ones I'm referring to are more modest and only about a half-inch thick. Shoulder pads add width to the upper body, taking some of the attention away from the lower half and giving a more balanced appearance.

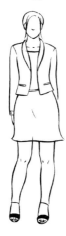

SHOULDER PADS HELP BALANCE OUT A PEAR-SHAPED BODY.

· If you have a small chest and a curvy bottom, padded bras are an option to produce a more proportioned look. If padded bras aren't your thing, don't sweat it; be natural.

· When searching for the perfect top, choose one that is looser fitting. Tight tops draw attention to your smaller upper body.

· Belts are a bit iffy, but if you must wear one, it should be on the narrow side.

· Don't wear pleats. In general, pleated skirts accentuate your curvy bottom, leaving you with a sort of pumpkin look.

· Bottom line on any side pockets: Don't be caught dead in them. That means: Goodwill, calling all cargo pants!

ARE YOU TOP-HEAVY?

If you've got a big chest and skinny hips and legs, you fall in this category. But that's not all bad!

Pluses and minuses

Top-heavy girls' pluses: A large chest (lucky you). Top-heavy girls' minuses: Your large chest can accentuate large shoulders, slim hips, and a flat butt. To bring more attention back to your face, follow these tips.

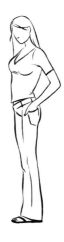

THE TOP-HEAVY FIGURE

What to do

- V-necks are best because they make your shoulders appear narrower, as well as showing off your cleavage (if that's the look you're going for). Other open necklines are also a possibility. If wearing a plunging neckline isn't appropriate, you could always wear a camisole underneath to cover what's necessary.

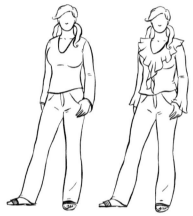

V-NECK TOPS ARE THE MOST FLATTERING
STYLE FOR TOP-HEAVY BODIES.
RUN FROM RUFFLES, FLOUNCES, AND
OTHER EXTRA DETAILS!

- Don't wear tops or jackets that have a lot of detail, like ruffles, patches, etc. All that extra detail adds more bulkiness to your upper body, making you appear even bigger.

- Never purchase jackets with shoulder pads (the opposite of pear-shaped girls). Remember, if it is big, it will add to your upper-body bulkiness.

- Longer tops are great because they help reduce the size of the chest (if that is what you prefer to do).

ARE YOU HIGH-WAISTED?

Determine whether you are high-waisted by trying on a pair of waist-high pants (if you still have a pair of those left in your closet!). If there is only about a 2-inch space between your breasts and your waist, you are definitely high-waisted.

Pluses and minuses

High-waisted girls' pluses: The length of your legs gives the impression of being tall. You lucky girl, you! Most of us would kill for your long legs! High-waisted girls' minuses: You have a shorter upper body.

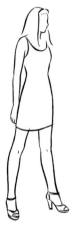

THE HIGH-WAISTED FIGURE

What to do

- To camouflage your high waist and give the impression of a lower waist, wear vertical patterns.

- V-necks, long necklaces, and extra-long scarves all help elongate your figure.

- Short vs. long tops: Don't wear short tops. They will accentuate your high waist. Instead, wear longer tops to give the illusion of a lower waistline.

- In general, belts set at the waist are a bad choice, because they shorten the upper body and draw attention to your high waist. Wear belts on your hips to camouflage where your true waistline is located, giving the illusion of a more evenly proportioned figure.

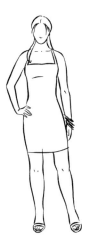

What to do
- Disguise where your true waistline is by having fun with layering. Layering is fashionable as well as 100 percent risk-free. When layering, be sure to always have the shorter layer on top.

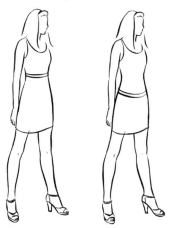

TO BALANCE A HIGH WAIST, WEAR YOUR BELTS AT THE HIPS, NOT AT THE WAIST.

ARE YOU LOW-WAISTED?

Determine whether you're low-waisted by trying on a pair of low-rise jeans or pants. If your upper body appears the same length between your head and the top of your waistband as from your waistband to your feet, you are more than likely low-waisted.

Pluses and minuses
Low-waisted girls' pluses: Due to the length of your upper body, most tops fit you better. Low-waisted girls' minuses: Often, your legs can appear shorter than they really are, making you look stubby.

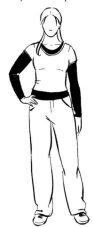

LAYERS DISGUISE A LOW WAIST.

- Narrow belts make your legs look longer. The wider your belt gets, the shorter your legs will appear.

- Don't wear capris and hip-huggers. Forget about pants that even give the impression of low riders. Bottom line: The lower the pant, the longer your upper body will look. The reason that lower pants give this impression is because they visually lower your waistline, making short legs appear even shorter. These styles of pants accentuate the length—or lack of length—of your legs.

- Miniskirts can make your legs look even shorter. If you are going to wear a skirt, the longer the skirt, the longer your legs will appear.

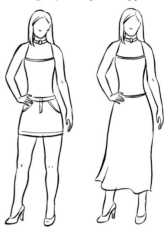

MINISKIRTS LOOK GREAT ON LONG-LEGGED GIRLS, BUT IF YOUR LEGS ARE SHORT, GO FOR LONGER SKIRTS.

- Heels coupled with pants will make your legs look long and supermodel-like.

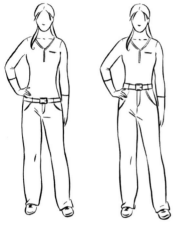

SEE HOW WEARING LOW-WAISTED PANTS MAKES YOUR LOW WAIST LOOK EVEN LOWER, WHILE HIGH-WAISTED PANTS MAKE YOUR FIGURE MORE BALANCED.

- High-waisted pants are the best style for you. The height of the waist will make your waist look higher, which will in turn make your legs look longer.

Ill-Fitting Attire

When was the last time that you went through your closet and purged? If it has been more than six months, I suggest that you go through and get rid of stuff that you haven't worn in at least two years. But before you get rid of everything, put it aside for a week and go through it again to make sure that you aren't getting rid of anything sentimental or something you could repurpose (refer to Chapter 6, Making Magic).

TOO BIG, TOO SMALL, TOO BAD

Your goal is to wear clothes that fit; they're always the most flattering. If you're not sure or are just in denial, here's how to tell when something looks good or if it needs to go.

You know it's too small when…

· Your tops create lines and pulling above and or between your boobs and are tight under the arms. It's a good idea to retire the shirt and either repurpose it or give it away to Goodwill.

· Shirts that ride up a little too much and too often while you're wearing them are too small. You may not feel like it's tight, but usually the fabric can't stay in place because it is being stretched too much.

· There are peepholes between your buttons, and you can see skin and/or your bra.

· Jeans and other thick-fabric pants are too small when there are horizontal lines that stretch across the crotch area. Another clue is when you have "camel toe." ("Camel toe" is when a pair of pants cuts in between your private parts.)

· This one may sound a little stupid, but sometimes we're in denial. If you can't sit down properly in a pair of pants without them being too tight and having an enormous roll popping over the edge, it's best to give them up.

You know it's too big when…

· Shirt sleeves should hit about 1 inch above your thumb knuckle. If shirt sleeves are longer than that, you can take advantage of it and cut thumbholes to keep your hands warm.

· A T-shirt, or any shirt that resembles a T-shirt, is too big if the neckline and armpits are hanging down. That is, unless the T-shirt is for working out or just lounging in.

· Halter tops that have separate triangles (or shaped) areas for your breast to fit in are too big when there are little open flaps near the armpits.

· Pants are too big if the crotch of the pants is 2 or more inches below your crotch (like guys' pants).

Other Figure Flaws

When it comes to reflecting upon ourselves, we are all so nitpicky. Here are a few tricks of the trade to hide or take attention away from the little things that bother us so much.

CHUNKY CALVES AND/OR "KANKLES"

"Kankles" are what you have when your ankle and calf give the appearance of being all one and undefined. Keep the attention away from these problem areas and direct the attention to other parts of your body. To do so, you must make a few sacrifices to avoid accentuating your calves and/or ankles.

· Tight pants and capri pants are definitely no-no's. Stay away from either of these styles. A combination of the two is lethal! Capri pants usually hit mid-calf, thus bringing attention to your calves or kankles.

- Miniskirts are also something to avoid. As far as longer skirts go, make sure that the skirt is floor-length. Skirts that aren't exactly floor-length tend to hit right at the ankles. This will accentuate your ankles, which is something you definitely do not want to do! If the skirt is ankle-length or above, consider wearing boots to cover the problem area.

- Boots with a thin (not stiletto) heel are a good choice. If you want to wear flats, flattering styles are usually shoes that have high-tops, like the Converse high-top or extra high-top, as well as Timberlands.

- Ankle-strap shoes and stilettos are also no-no's. Strappy shoes draw attention to the calves and ankles, which is exactly what you want to stay away from. Stilettos are no good because they will make your legs look bigger since the heels are so thin in comparison to your leg.

THE POUCH

Most of us girls have that little pouchy stomach that never seems to go away unless you're super-duper athletic or just blessed. One of my good friends, who wears a size 0, claims that even she has the "pouch." Bottom line is that most girls have it, and until you hit the gym and get an amazing six-pack I'll provide you with some tips on how to camouflage the pouch.

- Try shirts that aren't clingy (that doesn't necessarily mean baggy).

- Stay away from big, chunky belts unless you're wearing one over a loose-fitting tunic (or a loose, long shirt in general). Puff the tunic, or long shirt, over the belt slightly so that the shirt isn't entirely against your flesh.

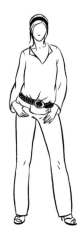

A TUNIC TOP IS A GREAT CAMOUFLAGE FOR "THE POUCH."

- Wearing pants that start right under the pouch is a bad idea. You will risk looking like you have a roll. It's best to stick with pants that either cover your pouch or are super low-cut, if you're daring.

Kiss My Precious Toes

When it comes to shoes, it can be said that shoes are a girl's second-best friend (diamonds are first). Every girl loves her shoes! With so many fabulous shoes out there to choose from, I want to help you pick the ones that are going to be flattering to your figure. That's right, shoes can be unflattering to your figure, and you didn't even know it!

SHOE PRECAUTIONS

Here are some shoes to avoid and some to go for. In some cases, a shoe style will look great on one type of leg and awful on another. So look in the mirror when you're trying them on! Look at your whole leg, not just the shoe. And choose shoes that make your legs look fantastic!

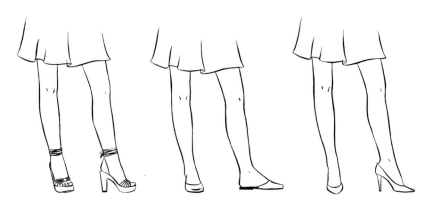

FLATS WITH A SLIGHT HEEL TEND TO MAKE EVERYONE'S LEGS LOOK LONGER, SO IF YOU'RE SHORT-LEGGED, THEY'RE THE WAY TO GO. AVOID CHUNKY HEELS IF YOUR LEGS ARE BIG OR THIN; THEY LOOK BEST ON MIDSIZE LEGS. STILETTOS LOOK FABULOUS ON TRIM LEGS BUT ACCENTUATE THE SIZE OF LARGER LEGS.

· Flats that have a slight heel will elongate your legs, which in turn will make you look taller. Slight heels are important in a low-waisted girl's wardrobe (see page 15).

· Soles that are on the thicker side usually look more like platforms, and everyone knows that those have been out of style ever since the Spice Girls.

· Although chunky heels are easier to walk on than thinner ones, consider this when purchasing chunky heels: The fat heel can make big legs look bigger and thin legs look scrawny. If you can't walk in thin heels, it's best to stick to flats or kitten heels (1- to 2-inch heels).

· The shoe you are wearing should be darker than your outfit. Plain black tennis shoes (with some accent color, like white) are something everyone should have in her closet, like the basic black Converse. Usually, plain black tennis shoes are an option for all outfits.

· On the other end of the spectrum, it's best to stay away from stilettos if your legs are a bit heavy. The heels being so thin will make your legs look even bigger. Stilettos are flattering on girls who have thin calves or just overall trim legs.

· Shoes that have really long straps that tie up your leg aren't really flattering on anyone. The reason is that to keep the shoe tied; you have to tie the straps really tight, thus creating diamond-shaped patches of skin oozing through.

· If you are one of those people who believes comfort should come before beauty, than the highest heel you should wear daily is 2 inches. Heels any higher than that aren't good for your feet.

"Okay, ladies. In this chapter, we've talked about what not to wear. In Chapter 2, It's Good for You, let's look at what we should be wearing!"

2. It's Good for You

Now it's time to talk about putting a look together, from the foundation up. From choosing the right bra to the secret of wearing stripes without looking fat, plus how to layer and accessorize, you'll find fashion advice that's good for you right here.

Underneath It All

Every outfit starts with a good foundation, and yes, ladies, that means we're talking about none other than bras and panties! Personally, I find bra and panty shopping to be the most fun! There are just so many styles, and there isn't a panty or bra that would be considered "unflattering." It's a win-win situation. Now you're probably curious what I'm going to write about after I just finished ranting and raving on both subjects. Well, read on and find out!

COME TO MY BOSOM...

The majority of us wind up wearing the wrong bra size. We don't consider that we've grown since the last visit to the mall for bras. It's best to be refitted every six months by a professional. At Victoria's Secret, for example, all the employees carry tape measures so they can quickly give you your bra size.

If you don't have time to go find out whether you're wearing the right bra size, you can always do the measurements yourself. For the band size, you measure just under your breast. For the cup size, you measure around

the fullest part of your breast and subtract the band size from the measure around the chest. Each inch is a cup size, so a 1-inch difference is an A, a 2-inch difference is a B, a 3-inch difference is a C, and a 4-inch difference is a D. For example: 34 inches (fullest part of breast) minus 32 inches (band size) equals a 2-inch difference, so that would mean you are a 32B.

Once you've found out your current size, make sure you wear the right style of bra under your clothing.

- Push-up bras are no good under snug-fitting high-neck tops. They will make you appear deformed.

- Lacy bras are pretty under thicker fabrics that don't show the texture of the lace through the fabric. For most tops, it's best to stick with a smooth, seamless bra.

- Underwire bras are my personal favorites. They are the best for support, especially if you are a size B or larger.

- Shaped push-up bras are an option for girls who have small chests and wouldn't mind some extra "umph." Victoria's Secret has a great push-up, padded bra with convertible straps, so you can wear it with tube tops, halters, or normal sleeves.

- Side-padded bras are great if you just want a little extra cleavage.

DEDICATION TO THE THONG

The right choice of underwear is basic to all fabulous-looking outfits. Without it, your pants or skirt can look tacky from underwear lines or look bad if your underwear bunches up in the back. Also, the unsightly underwear lines make indentations in your butt, making it look fat—and not in the good rap-music-video-girl way, either. That is why thongs are simply the best! Thongs give that no-pantyline look under everything you wear. Thongs take a little getting used to, but don't be threatened by the string that happens to fit in between your butt cheeks: It really isn't uncomfortable.

TEXTURE-IZE ME, CAPTAIN

One way to make single color dressing interesting is by adding texture to the mix. For example, you could wear a combination of velour, satin, thermal, wool, denim, jersey, suede, cashmere (if it's affordable), ribbing, terry cloth, or tweeds—not all of those together, of course! Imagine a terry cloth running suit with a denim jacket, a ribbed tank, and some suede boots. This outfit would be extremely cute in tones of blue with a hint of color in the boots (like a neutral color), and the tank could be white. It's simple but very intricate due to the differences in texture.

SINGLE-COLOR COORDINATING

If you want to look taller or thinner, try wearing an outfit that's all the same color (or shades of that color). Think basic black. I'm not saying that you should wear the same shade all the time: You would wind up looking like a giant blueberry if you were wearing navy blue or like a string bean if you wore all the same shade of green. Good one color dressing means wearing different textures and/or shades of the same color. A celebrity who pulls this off well is Raven Symone from the television show *That's So Raven* on the Disney Channel.

If you're serious about dressing in a single color, it's best to stick with dark shades. (Picture this: A bright red ensemble would do nothing but make you look ultra-bright, Santa-like, and extremely fashion-ignorant.) To pull off the look, the fundamental parts of your outfit, i.e. your top and bottom, should be the same color.

Combining pieces of the same color but different textures helps add interest while still providing the slimming/ lengthening effect.

Yikes! Stripes!

Most girls tend to stay away from stripes, because they've been warned that stripes make you look wider. One of the most common misconceptions is that all stripes make you look bigger. That is untrue: Vertical stripes actually make you look taller and thinner. Of course, it's pretty much an illusion.

Don't beat yourself up about looking bad in horizontal stripes. My math teacher has showed us many illusions, and you know it's a trick of your eyes and mind, but when it comes to ourselves, we often forget that.

If you want to try stripes for yourself, read these rules before heading to the mall:

· The wider the space between stripes, the wider you will appear.

· Vertical stripes on clingy fabrics are no-no's, because once the garment is on, it will curve to the contours of your body, making you look wider.

· Diagonal lines are flattering. Try shirts that have crisscross necklines. They will bring attention up toward your face and accentuate your cleavage, as well as lengthening your body.

· The only time that horizontals will really work is if they're between your chest and your waist. A great example is the line of tube dresses/shirts that Juicy sold in 2003–2004.

Layering

Layering adds a lot to an outfit. It gives it another dimension as well as making it look more interesting. Layering can also provide a "buffer zone" that steers attention away from your tummy. Here are some tips on how to layer the best possible way:

· The way to make the layers look best is to choose two lightweight shirts that are approximately the same design. The heavier the shirts, the bulkier you will appear.

· The bottom layer should be fitted and longer than the top layer.

· If you are concerned about drawing attention to your "pouch" (see page 18 for more on this), choose similar colors for both layers.

· If you want to wear a cropped jacket, wear a longer shirt. This look is best on girls who aren't pear-shaped.

· Camisoles are an option for the top layer, while men's "wife beaters" (since they are longer than little-boy "wife beaters") are always an option for the bottom layer.

HOT TIP

Layering is a great way to make your outfit more appealing. Make sure that the darker layer is always the bottom layer. Sometimes doing it reversed can look good depending on the color of the bottoms you are wearing.

SCARVES

You're probably wondering how scarves could be included in the layering section. Well, scarves add another layer to an otherwise basic outfit. Here's what to do with them:

· Thin scarves as well as thicker scarves (ones that will actually keep you warm in cold weather) are options for obscuring your tummy by leaving the scarf wrapped around your neck and having it hang down under an open jacket. If you don't have the "tire" (the fat that accumulates around your hips, lower back, and tummy), you could always lose the jacket and just wear a light-weight scarf.

· There are three acceptable ways to wear scarves. Option one, wrap the scarf around your neck and have it draped in front of you. Option two, wear the scarf around your neck and have it draped behind you. Option three, hold both ends of the scarf with one hand to make a really oblong U, then take that and put it around your neck (like you would a towel) and put the non-looped end through the little U loop. Please, no movie star scarf-wraps around the head.

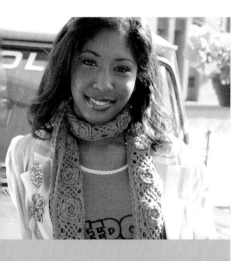

Accessories

They say that your accessories can either make or break your outfit. In this section, I will give you guidelines on good accessory choices versus bad accessory choices.

BELTS

Belts are a great way to add to an outfit. When purchasing a belt, there are a few ground rules that will help you determine which belts are the better buy.

· Invest in an upscale, versatile belt to make any outfit miraculously look expensive.

· It's best to buy a belt that is a little big so you can have the option of wearing it on your waist or lower on your hips (see page 78).

· When hooking a belt, there should always be about an inch of the belt going through the belt loop. Otherwise, even if the belt fits fine, it will give the illusion that you are bigger.

· When wearing a belt over a baggy T-shirt or tunic, wear the belt on your hips and have it a little loose so that it will slant to one side.

· It's not only important to look cute from the front, but it's also important to look good from the back. Instead of buckling your belt in the front like always, consider moving the buckle to the back over either butt cheek.

· Chain belts are always great, but make sure that you don't wear them with knits because you'll wind up ruining the knit as well as being stuck to yourself.

· When not wearing your belts, hang them on hooks or roll them and store them in a basket or drawer.

HATS

Most people know whether they can "pull off" hats or not. If you're one of those people who just doesn't look good in hats, don't take it personally, but feel free to move on to the jewelry section (page 26).

Although it might not seem like there is a certain way to wear different styles of hats, there is. I will provide you with tips for wearing different styles more stylishly.

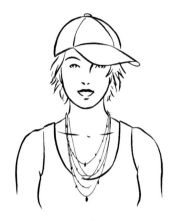

BASEBALL CAP/TRUCKER HAT

· The baseball cap/trucker hat is best worn either straight, with the bill pointing forward, or slightly shifted to one side, so that it is noticeably off center, but not completely to the side.

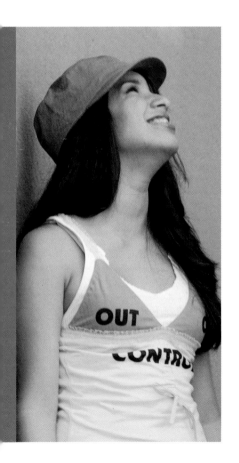

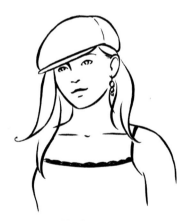

DRIVER CAP

· Driver caps are best worn straight, with the bill pointing forward and slightly pulled down to cover your eyes. Don't pull down the hat too low, because you should still be able to see properly without tipping your head up.

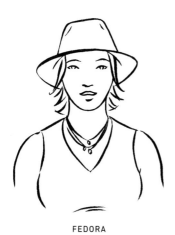

FEDORA

· Fedoras, like the classic hat Alicia Keys often wears, are best worn like she wears it, slightly to one side and pulled down low over the eyes. That way it kind of gives off the mysterious vibe.

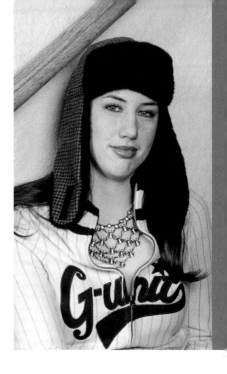

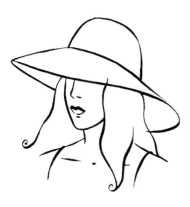

BIG FLOPPY HAT

· Big floppy hats are best worn if part of the brim is covering one eye, and one eye only, but for the most part, floppy hats aren't that practical.

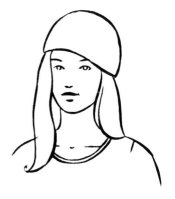

BEANIE

· Bucket hats and beanies are pretty much self-explanatory; there really is no special way to wear them besides simply putting it on. As for beanies with brims, those are best worn like you would wear a base-ball cap.

JEWELRY

Your jewelry can be what really makes your outfit—or breaks it. These tips will help you make your jewelry work for you, not against you.

- Silver versus gold: Generally speaking, if you're wearing one, don't wear the other at the same time.

- Long necklaces are great. They make a vertical statement, creating length and height. Try wrapping a necklace around your neck twice to create a choker and leaving an abundance of the strand hanging.

- Thick chokers can make you look like you have a short neck. Wear them if you like them, but remember that thinner is better than wider, unless you have a "giraffe neck."

- Bigger-boned girls should stay away from smaller pieces of jewelry because they will make their bodies look bigger.

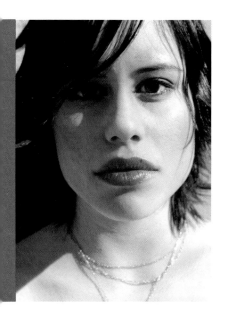

- Brooches always look better grouped with other brooches instead of being worn individually. The same goes for bracelets and rings. However, you shouldn't wear more than three brooches at a time.

- When purchasing earrings, it's always important to remember quality and not quantity. I prefer dangling earrings to studs, but that's personal preference.

PURSES

Clothing styles and fabrics are very specific when it comes to the different seasons—winter, fall, spring, and summer —as well as casual versus party styles. Purses, on the other had, aren't quite as specific. Purses can be pretty much mixed and matched with any season, with the exception of wearing a fur bag during summer or spring or wearing a pastel purse in the fall or winter.

For health purposes, it's best to stick with a small- to medium-size bag, because the bigger the bag, the more room there is to put things. It is proven that if you wear a heavy purse on one shoulder, over time that shoulder will become slightly lower. You might also put out your shoulder carrying a heavy bag over time. Backpacks, however, balance the weight between both shoulders.

Handbags are always at a flattering length, but personally I prefer over-the-shoulder bags so that I can have my hands free. The length of the strap is a little trickier. If you have a wide hip and stomach area, avoid strap lengths that will make the purse hit at your hips. Instead, go for a bag that will wind up under your arm. On the other end of the spectrum, if you're really tall, ultra-long straps will give you the illusion of being slightly shorter.

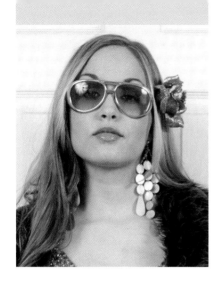

- Oval faces look good in almost every lens shape.

- Square faces (sharp jawline and same width across temples, cheekbones, and jawline) look best in rounded lenses.

- Triangular (full cheekbones and jawline, pointy chin) and heart-shaped faces (wide forehead and cheekbones, narrower jawline) look best with lenses that extend toward the cheeks.

- Round faces look best with squarish lenses.

SUNGLASSES

Sunglasses are a great accessory, and they bring attention directly to your face. But sunglasses, unlike other accessories, can only be worn at certain times without looking ridiculous. Sunglasses are suitable only for daylight wear and being outdoors. At all other times, skip the sunglasses. Clearish lenses are the only exception to the don't-wear-sunglasses-indoors rule.

The shape of the sunglasses should be complementary to the shape of your face. There isn't really any right or wrong style of sunglasses for your face, though. The only way to really tell whether the sunglasses look good on you is by trying them on and judging for yourself. However, there are a few little-known tips that should help you choose which sunglasses to try on:

TIGHTS

Although tights seem like something that should only be worn with fancy dresses, tights happen to spice up an outfit when you're wearing either torn jeans or miniskirts. When wearing a pair of tights with a miniskirt, it's best to stick with a slightly translucent fabric. Also, try cutting off the bottom part of your tights, making them mid-calf length. When it comes to wearing tights under ripped pants, depending on where the rips are, you could wear a range of translucent as well as opaque tights. Patterned tights always look good under a pair of ripped jeans.

"So, now that you know what looks good, what about shopping? Well, that's what the next chapter is all about…"

3. Before Hitting the Road

Before you head out on your next shopping spree or casual window-shopping adventure, there are a few things that you should keep in mind to keep yourself on track. It's always best to draw up a list of things that you're looking for. It doesn't mean that you have to get everything on your list; it will just help you keep your eyes open for those specific things.

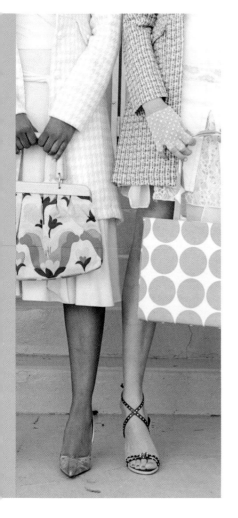

Sales Smarts

Everyone loves a good sale. When someone asks you where you got something, it's always so rewarding to say, "I got it from _____, on sale!" Then usually the other person is like, "Really?" and she winds up thinking you're this terrific shopper, and la-di-da! The trick is how to find the sales when it isn't the day after Thanksgiving or Christmas. One way is to ask. Department stores sometimes have one-day-only special unadvertised sales (see "My Cool Sale Coup" on page 29). Next time you're in a favorite store, ask the sales staff whether and when there's going to be one.

MY COOL SALE COUP

At Macy's department stores, they have this sale that is on random Sundays, called Door Buster sales, and you get an additional percentage off things that are already marked down. These sales go from the time Macy's opens in the morning until 1:00 in the afternoon. These Door Buster sales aren't posted anywhere, so when you go into Macy's to do your shopping, ask a salesperson when the next one will be.

I have a great story about one of these Door Buster sales that happened just a few months ago. Every time I went into Macy's, I saw these four handbags from Fetish by Eve. I really wanted one, but they were $144 each—I couldn't afford it. (My mom knew how much I loved those purses; she was secretly planning on getting me one as a present for doing well in school.) Every time I was in Macy's, I stood there admiring them and contemplating whether I should just splurge. I wound up not getting them, and I felt remorse about not purchasing them.

Well, one Sunday when my mom was going to get me the purse, I went with her into Macy's and they were having their Door Buster sale. I checked the handbag section of the store, and the Fetish purses were on sale and marked down even more because of the sale. I wound up getting all four of the purses for less than the price of one! Patience really does pay.

Another important factor in finding good sales is checking the newspapers. Usually, department stores and larger chains will have extra-percentage-off coupons in the newspaper. If you don't have time to make it to a newspaper and find a coupon, you should always ask when ringing up your purchased items. The salespeople aren't out to get you; they will use the coupon that they have on hand for when customers ask. Don't be intimidated; the worst that will happen is that there isn't a sale, and oh well.

Sales at boutiques or small chains are a little harder to detect. It's best to check in at the changing of the seasons; usually things go on sale then. It's always nice to keep returning to a boutique, because you can develop a relationship with the employees, and they can give you a heads up on when the next sale is going to be. For example, in Los Angeles, there is a street called Melrose, and there are a ton of boutiques there. These boutiques are great because whenever you go, the same people are always working there. Last word when it comes to boutiques: Don't be fooled; not all boutiques are super expensive.

Upscale stores like Guess and Bebe are usually beyond the budget of the average teenage girl. But don't be too intimidated to go into these stores! It's always good to pop in, because they often do have sale racks in the back of their stores with incredibly cute things marked down. A reminder when it comes to designer garments on sale: Just because it's designer and marked down does not mean that you should buy it. Even if there's nothing on sale (or nothing that appeals to you), consider trips to designer stores to be good scouting expeditions. You can check out the hot looks and maybe come up with your own affordable versions.

If you're located in a metropolitan city, such as New York City or Los Angeles, there is a garment district where there are tons of great finds for inexpensive prices. Usually you can get an even better price than what's marked on the tag, as well as avoid paying sales tax.

HOT TIP

Often in the heat of big sales, we ladies tend to buy anything and everything that appears to be halfway decent. In the midst of digging through sale merchandise, it's best to think of it as if it were full price. Don't think in terms of "For $10, I'll buy it!" Look at the original price, and if you would still buy it at that price, then chances are that you probably really do like it. Just because something is marked down doesn't mean you love it. Remember: When it comes to buying anything, you must love it, no exceptions!

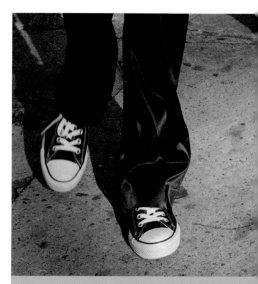

Keeping Tags and Receipts

Tags and receipts are something that you should keep all the way up until you actually wear the piece. Returning things at department stores or clothing-store chains is quite simple: Usually all you have to do is bring back the piece with the receipts and tags intact within thirty days, and you'll get your money back. (You get a store credit if you don't have the receipts.)

It's best to keep all clothing that you've recently purchased in the bag that you bought it in, with the receipts. This way, you have a visual reminder that you haven't worn it, and if you do happen to change your mind on the piece, you have it already stowed in a bag, with the receipts. And you can check the bag daily to see whether you really do like the piece enough to wear it within the first two weeks of purchasing it—that is, unless the weather or occasion prohibits it.

Boutiques are a little harder to return clothes to. Some boutiques do allow returns for up to ten days, but normally, boutiques only give store credit, even if you do return something within the ten days. To be safe, you should be 100 percent sure upon purchasing that you really want that particular piece.

Once you get a piece home, you should try it on again just to make sure that you like the fit of something. Sometimes the lighting and mirrors in clothing stores can give false perceptions of certain garments. After you have tried your new treasure on at home and are going to wear it out that day (or night), you can finally cut off the tags.

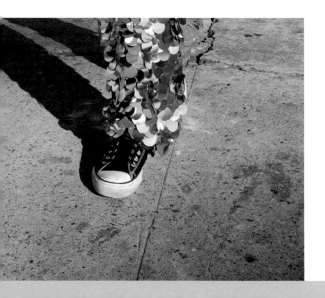

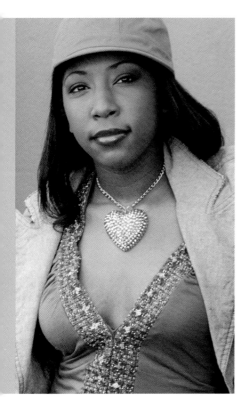

Taking Care of Your Stuff

Most of the time, you probably get rid of clothing because it's worn out, it's old, or you just don't wear it anymore. But if you take care of your clothing, you can preserve things for a long time while simultaneously making them look better. For example, no one wants to wear a "pillie" top. Pilling makes the top look old even if you've worn it only once. To prevent shirts from pilling, you should keep them away from rough surfaces, wash them inside out, and line-dry them. That means don't put them in the dryer, but instead, hang them somewhere to dry; this also prevents shrinking. You can buy special drying racks that are made for drying clothes. They have a series of places to hang your clothes so they can dry.

The bottom line when it comes to anything that has rhinestones, crystals, sequins, embroidery, or any detail whatsoever: It's best to wash it inside out by hand or on a delicate machine wash, or, if it's affordable, have it dry-cleaned. If you opt for dry cleaning, look in your local papers for dry-cleaning discount coupons. The money you save could go toward buying something new.

HOT TIP

Getting stuff dry-cleaned is a pain, not to mention expensive. Keep your dry-cleaning bill down by washing some dry-clean-only pieces by hand or on the gentle cycle in the washing machine. Line-dry after washing. (Never wash cashmere, silk, or wool; always dry-clean them.)

There are always those accidental times when you rip clothing or break an accessory. When it comes to rips, they are usually easy to fix if the rip is located on the seam. In that case, turn the piece inside out and sew on the seam with a needle and thread, or, if you know how to use a sewing machine, you could throw a few stitches in that way. If the tear is somewhere besides the seam, see whether you can possibly repurpose the piece by either covering the rip with a patch or cutting even more to make it look like you did it on purpose. If that doesn't work, then it's best to retire the piece and just mark it down as a loss.

Stains on clothing, such as blood, rust, grass stains, or nail polish, can usually be removed by a product called Folex. This is a miracle stain remover that even works if the stain is already set, although it is best to put Folex on the stain as soon as possible.

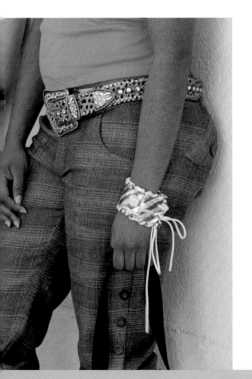

FIXING BROKEN ACCESSORIES

Jewelry is a tad harder to fix than clothes, since you usually need tools. Here are some handy-dandy ways to fix your jewelry:

· Most of the time when jewelry breaks, it's because the little O-ring that connects the piece somewhere is loose. When this happens, you can get some pliers and use them to clinch the O-ring shut and, voilà, your piece is fixed. This applies mostly to earrings, necklaces, and bracelets.

· If there is a metal chain involved and it happens to break, you can go to a craft store and pick up a replacement chain. If you don't want to hassle with a metal chain, you could use a suede string or piece of ribbon.

· If you have a ring that falls apart, meaning the pretty part falls off of the band, you can glue the pretty part back onto the ring with E6000 glue that you can purchase at a craft shop.

The only way to keep sunglasses from breaking and scratching is to keep them in a case. When you buy glasses, you'll normally receive a case, but if you don't, you could always ask for one. If you don't have a case, and don't have the time to pick one up, you could always use a pouch or sock to put your glasses in to keep them from getting scratched.

Hats don't so much break as get squished. Hats with a shape, such as fedoras (see page 25), can be mounted on other hats of the same shape. Avoid squishing the hats with other things, because this will make the hats lose their shape.

Take-Away Tips

I know I've told you some of these before, but here's a handy checklist of my favorite tips. Read them before putting an outfit together or heading to the mall—or copy the list and take it with you!

· Before giving away old clothing, look to see whether there is anything you could repurpose.

· Anything you purchase, you must love!

· Check the newspaper before going to the mall; you could find sales and an additional percentage off.

· When at the checkout counter, ask yourself, "Is this worth every penny?"

· Don't buy in haste: Chances are, you will wear it once and it will then be forgotten.

· When wearing a shirt that has a high neckline, don't wear a necklace, unless the necklace is really long.

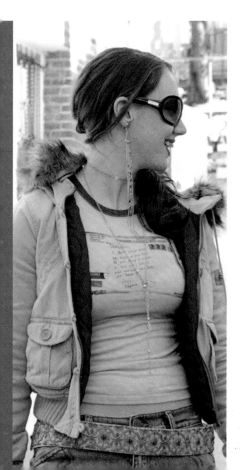

- Denim is very important in a wardrobe. Having a lot of jeans in all different styles is a good idea.

- Your shoes should always be darker than the rest of your outfit. Normally, it's hard to pull off white shoes.

- Tight & Tight: Stay away from wearing a tight top and a tight bottom; you'll look "cheap."

- When your feet have stopped growing, it's a good idea to invest a little more money in your shoes. Higher quality shoes will look better and last longer.

- When putting together an outfit, not everything has to be in matching colors, but the colors do have to complement each other.

- The higher your heels, the longer your skirt should be.

- If pants are too long and you don't have the time to sew them under, use a bobby pin. Fold the pants leg to the length you want and secure it by using a bobby pin in the front and back of each leg.

- Tying a shirt up in the back to make it a crop top is tacky. If the shirt is already cropped, that's not tacky.

- Cheap & Cheap: Generally, wearing several inexpensive pieces will make the whole outfit look inexpensive. My suggestion is to invest in a few key items that are a little on the more expensive side (whatever you can afford), and mix them with other pieces that are less expensive to give the whole outfit a very chic look.

- Remember: When purchasing something, it should look as good if not better on you than on the hanger.

- Creating different outfits is a way to express yourself.

- Fashion should be fun—not frustrating!

"Ready to shop yet? Not so fast, ladies! Before you head out the door, read the Ten Clothing Commandments starting on the next page."

4. The Ten Clothing Commandments: The "Rules" for Your Fashion Creation

There's just one more thing you should know before you head out to shop and drop—my Ten Clothing Commandments. Follow these ten little rules for fashion success—and to avoid serious shopping disasters! You'll see how my friends and I learned them the hard way, so you don't have to...

The First Clothing Commandment

Thou shall not hoard all the shopping meccas to thyself.

When it comes to great shopping, it's better to share the wealth. Sometimes the little devil standing on your shoulder tries to get the best of you and keeps you from telling your friends. I would never have known some of the best stores and boutiques existed if I hadn't learned about them through my friends. Bottom line, you give your friends the information on good shopping, they'll reciprocate (hopefully). If you're worried about your friends copying your style, just remember that copying is the highest form of flattery!

The Second Clothing Commandment

Thou shall not leave thy clothing and shoes lying about.

For most girls, it's usually a pain to hang up their clothes, fold things, and put their shoes away. It's so much easier to leave your clothing and shoes lying around your room. Who really cares? Let me tell you: There are a lot more reasons for you to clean up your clothes then there are reasons against it. First of all, it doesn't take too much time to put dirty clothes in a laundry bin and hang and fold clean clothes. (Putting the clothes in drawers and your closet, well, that's a different story, especially if they're messy.) The perks for keeping your clothing hung or folded are that you won't find any mysterious stains appearing; your clothing won't be wrinkled; your shoes will keep a better shape; and overall, everything will last longer. If you have animals, especially cats, you'd better be equipped with a lint roller at all times, especially for your darks.

A FELINE FIASCO

It wasn't too long ago that I left a pair of shoes lying on the ground instead of putting them away in my closet. Well, let's just say I learned my lesson. When I went back to where those shoes were, just as I was about to slip my foot in, I saw a clump of cat barf! I was horror-stricken: My cat barfed in my shoe! Luckily, I saw it before I stepped in it. Moral: Don't leave your shoes (or clothing, for that matter) lying around; they might be barfed on, or worse!

The Third Clothing Commandment

Thou shall not borrow thy neighbor's clothes.

A lot of girls I know borrow each other's clothes. They always promise each other that they will return it soon, but it usually takes weeks, if not months, before the girl gets the thing she leant back. Bottom line, it's best not to borrow clothes, because it can end a friendship or at least deteriorate a friendship, especially if it was something that was a favorite of yours and was damaged. The only exception is if you are going to lend something to a girlfriend and she'll return it that night, because you are there with her to remind her. Otherwise, say no.

The Fourth Clothing Commandment

Thou shall not purchase, wear, and return.

It's not good or nice to purchase, wear, and return. Either you like it enough to keep it or you don't like it enough so you return it. In the interim, don't just wear it for the sake of wearing it. Usually, cotton shirts tend to stretch a little bit after being worn for a long period of time, such as a school day. Plus, how would you feel if you found out that someone wore a garment once or even twice before you bought it? Even if the previous occupier didn't leave any visual damage, it still doesn't feel good to wear. It would almost be like purchasing used clothing, except you're paying full price.

The Fifth Clothing Commandment

Thou shall not betray thy lady friend and tell her that she looks good in something that looks heinous.

When it comes to shopping with friends, we don't want to be mean, but sometimes things just don't look flattering, plain and simple. The worst thing you could do is tell a friend that she looks good in something that really doesn't fit her well. Not only will this make you feel guilty later, but a friend of yours is going to be wearing something ugly out and about. That doesn't mean you have to break the news to her meanly. You could say, "I don't think that it looks that flattering." Or, "I liked that other shirt you tried on before better." This way, you won't feel bad in the end, and even if your friend can't appreciate your opinion at that moment, she will eventually realize that you are an honest friend.

UNFRIENDLY ADVICE

A friend of my mom's found out years later that her best friend told her she looked good when in fact she looked terrible. It was devastating to her, even though she was a grown woman when she found out. She said that to this day it still hurts her feelings. Her "best friend" who deceived her admitted that she did so out of jealousy. Moral· You can admire a friend for what she has, but don't do nasty things out of jealousy, because then you really aren't her friend.

The Sixth Clothing Commandment

Thou shall only purchase what thou truly loves.

One thing that a lot of girls do—I do this myself—is buy things in haste. For example, you will go shopping and not really find anything that you want to buy, and all of a sudden, you find something halfway decent and decide that you're getting it just because you don't have anything to wear to school that week. These purchases are bad because you probably will wind up hardly ever wearing the piece, and you will feel crappy later and often ask yourself, "Why did I buy this to begin with?" That's why it's best to be in love with everything you purchase. This way, your money won't go to waste, and you will absolutely love everything in your closet.

HOW I LEARNED TO BUY WHAT I LOVE AND LOVE WHAT I BUY

When I was younger and my mom still paid for everything, I used to choose things to buy and never wear them. My mom got fed up with my purchasing things that I never wore, so she made me buy my own clothing by giving me an allowance. This taught me to think twice before I bought something, and it made me realize that I must love it!

The Seventh Clothing Commandment

Thou shall not spend all thy clothing allowance on fads.

A big mistake that girls make is when they spend all their clothing allowance on the latest fad. Most of my friends who do this usually cover up by saying that they'll wear it even when the fad is out because they like it. This never happens. Ugg boots have been a major fad the past two years. One of my friends bought pretty much every color of the Ugg boots; now that this fad is fading, she doesn't know what to do with all of them. This example shows that you can buy into fads moderately, but don't get carried away.

The Eighth Clothing Commandment

Thou shall not wear the same outfit to the same place in a three-week rotation period.

By mixing and matching, you should be able to create a three-week rotation period or more with your wardrobe. You can achieve this by layering your tops, adding accessories, wearing different shoes or jackets, and adding a scarf or a hat. You should get lots of ideas on mixing and matching from the rest of this book!

The Ninth Clothing Commandment

Thou shall not buy anything that is not thy right size, even if thou loves it.

Just because you really want something and they don't have your size still doesn't give you the right to purchase it. I know in Commandment Six I said that you should buy only what you love—but only if they have your correct size! If you buy something too small, it will be uncomfortable and look bad. Shirts that are too big usually look bad because they don't fit

correctly, unless it's a T-shirt. I suggest that if you really love something, and they don't have your size, you should either check on the store's Web site or ask when they are going to be getting another shipment in and give them your contact information as well as your size. You should always follow up in a day or two.

WHEN HER LOSS WAS MY GAIN
One of my mom's clients really wanted this pair of snakeskin Prada flats, but they didn't have her size; she bought them anyway a half-size too small. Well, she found them uncomfortable, and now those Prada shoes reside in my closet! (At least one of us is happy!)

The Tenth Clothing Commandment

Thou shall take care of thyself.

When you take care of yourself, like your hair, skin, teeth, and body, you will make your outfits look better. Instead of your clothes wearing you, you will be wearing your clothes.

"Remember to read these Ten Clothing Commandments over again before you shop—you'll be glad you did! Now, turn the page, and you can find out how I put a look together."

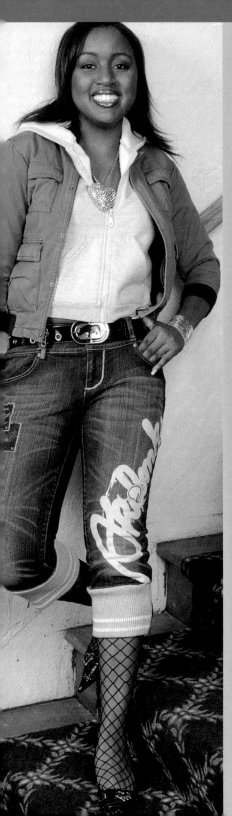

Part Two : How to Put an Outfit Together

5. How I Do What I Do

Many times people say to me, "I love your outfit! I would have never thought to put that together, how did you come up with that?" Unfortunately, there isn't a cookie-cutter way to come up with an outfit. It normally happens through trial and error.

Sometimes I am inspired by something I see a celebrity wearing. Back in 2002, before trucker hats were popular, I saw Eve wear one on MTV. I was inspired, and went out to Target the next day and picked up a trucker hat from the men's department. When I wore the trucker hat to school, all of my friends made fun of me and told me I looked like a wannabe gardener. Lo and behold, the next thing that everyone knew, trucker hats were the "it" thing. I guess I was just before my time!

Design Around a Favorite Piece

Another way that I get ideas for an outfit is when I know what particular piece I want to wear. For example, I went to the mall for the after-Christmas sale. In Bebe, there were these great brown sweats that could be made into an ultra-fashionable outfit or just casual wear for the gym. When I got home, I laid those sweats on my bed and picked out about five different shirts that I thought would look good with them. I narrowed it down to two, and I tried on both shirts with the pants. It just so happened that both shirts looked great with the pants, so I had two new outfits. I just added shoes and accessories to go with each one.

You could use this technique with pretty much anything that you're thinking about wearing. Usually, the more layers to the outfit, the more fashionable it will appear. I'm not saying that you should keep layering until you can't move and you look like a snowman, but just that it looks nice if you have double-layer shirts and a jacket, and possibly a scarf if it's cold.

Dressing for the Weather and the Occasion

It's also important to keep in mind that you should dress in a style that's weather-appropriate. At my school (I go to Beverly Hills High School, if you're curious), there are a lot of girls who still wear skirts even if the temperature is in the 60s and dropping. Although some of their outfits are cute and just wouldn't look as good with pants, it looks ridiculous and takes away from how good they could look if they were wearing something warm, given the temperature. Bottom line: Don't get hypothermia during the winter for the sake of a skirt and don't get heat stroke during the summer for the sake of layering! I would say comfort first, but I like high heels, and I don't think that those will ever be "comfortable"—only tolerable.

Another aspect to keep in mind is making sure that what you wear is appropriate for the occasion. Freshman year, I thought it was genius to wear heels every day to school. My feet got used to it, but this year I retired my heels for school wear and now reserve them for the weekends. It's best to wear flats to school or, if you must, kitten heels. Leave high heels for the weekends.

When dressing for school, be casual; don't look like you are about to go to the club, even if the outfit is hot. Make sure that you look like someone who's going to school. As far as fancier occasions go, I would say that if it isn't too fancy, you could get by in a pair of nice jeans, heels, and a blazer or some other upscale jacket. If there are going to be a lot of adults, or the majority of the people are adults, refrain from showing too much cleavage. I'm sure that all the 30-, 40-, and 50-year-olds wouldn't appreciate looking at a teenager's boobs!

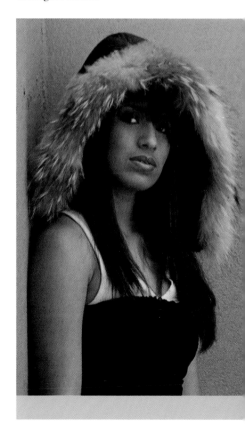

Mixing and Matching

When it comes to mixing and matching, remember that not every piece of an outfit has to match exactly the color of the other parts of the outfit. You could always wear complementary colors. On New Year's, I wore a Lakers purple top with jeans and fuchsia and pink jewelry. The fuchsia and pink were complementary colors to the Lakers' purple. Think about mixing your own colors; experiment and have fun! After all, it doesn't really take any talent to match the same color up with itself. If you are interested in mixing colors, you could try mixing:

- Wine red with all shades of brown
- Coral with yellows, light greens, turquoises, pinks, or oranges
- Purple with greens, pinks, or blues
- Blues with pinks, oranges, yellows, or some greens
- Pinks with blues, oranges, purples, corals, or greens

See what combinations look good to you—and on you!

Express Yourself!

If you're ever unsure about an outfit, you could always try asking a girl-friend, sister, or your mother. They will tell you the truth—whether they like it or not. But if you really like an outfit and other people tell you that they don't like it, don't stop yourself from wearing it for the sake of others.

Fashion is a way to express yourself, so don't confine yourself to a trend or what others want you to wear. Fashion is something you can have fun and experiment with. The best advice I can give you when it comes to creating outfits is to be open-minded and go crazy. Usually, you'll come up with something fabulous, while simultaneously turning heads.

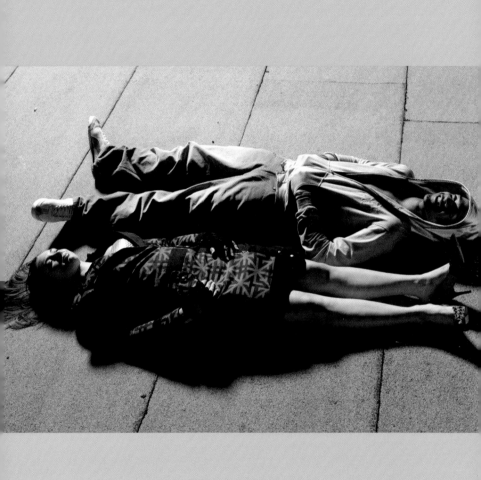

6. Making Magic

When we find a fashion item we really love, whether it is a piece of jewelry, a purse, sunglasses, clothing, or sometimes even shoes, we never stop and think that we could possibly make it on our own.

Or maybe you do think that you could make something, but you just don't know exactly how to go about it. Well, in this chapter, I'll share a variety of different things you can make.

Maybe you won't want to copy my exact examples, but instead apply the techniques to your own ideas or needs. Whatever the case, be creative, have fun, and don't be afraid to make mistakes—although it is best to start working on something that doesn't have much value to you!

Below you will find a scale that will measure the difficulty level of each project. Decide whether you're a novice, intermediate, or experienced by reading each project to see how hard or easy it looks to you. If you haven't made or done anything of this sort before, or did a terrible job last time you tried, then you're probably a novice; if you have attempted something like the projects listed below and they turned out decent, you're intermediate; if you have tried more than one of these projects and mastered them beautifully then you are, no doubt, experienced. If you are either intermediate or experienced, you can also work on projects that are lower than your experience level.

DIFFICULTY	SYMBOL
Novice	★
Intermediate	★★
Experienced	★★★

CUT-UP CLOTHES

All the projects in this section involve cutting clothes to make them more stylish. You'll need the same equipment to do them all (see "What You Will Need," below), plus the piece of clothing (T-shirt, jeans, sweatshirt, or whatever it is) that you're cutting. So collect these in your work space before you start.

WHAT YOU WILL NEED:

Scissors

Flat surface to cut on

Ruler

Pencil

Knots Down the Back

Difficulty: ★★

WHAT YOU WILL NEED:

T-shirt

Flat surface to cut on

Ruler

Pencil

Scissors

KEEP IN MIND: Use a loose-fitted T-shirt. And don't make the knots so tight that you can't fit in the shirt!

WHAT TO DO:

1. Lay the T-shirt you want to cut down on a flat, hard surface, with the back of the shirt facing up.

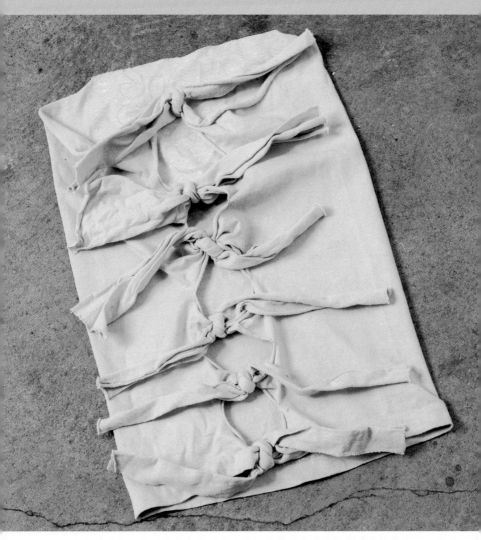

2. Take your ruler and pencil and make a straight line from the neckline all the way down to the bottom of the shirt.

3. Use your scissors to cut along the line. (Make sure you only have one layer of fabric in your hand.)

4. Fold the shirt on its side so that one shoulder is facing up.

5. Hold the recently cut part of the shirt (both layers) in one hand, and with the other hand cut horizontal slits (about 2 inches long and 1 to 3 inches apart) all the way from the neckline to the bottom of the shirt.

6. Unfold the shirt and lay it back down on the table facing up.

7. You should see a whole bunch of T-shirt fringe (big, chunky, rectangular pieces on either side).

8. Start to tie and double-knot each rectangular piece of fabric with its mate across from it.

9. Once you have tied the knots all the way down the back, go back to each knot and slightly pull on the fabric surrounding it, in order to make the knots tighter and show a little more skin.

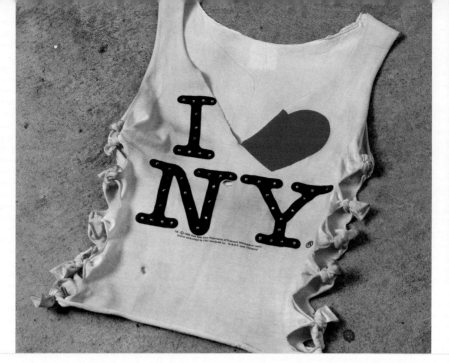

Knots Down the Sides

Difficulty: ★★

WHAT YOU WILL NEED:

T-shirt

Flat surface to cut on

Ruler

Pencil

Scissors

KEEP IN MIND: Use a loose-fitted T-shirt. And don't make the knots so tight that you can't fit in the shirt!

WHAT TO DO:

1. Lay the T-shirt on its side on a flat surface, with one shoulder facing up.

2. Fold the sleeve up. Take your ruler and pencil and draw a straight line from under the armpit all the way to the bottom of the shirt. (You can skip this step if your shirt has a seam down the side.)

3. Use your scissors to cut along the line. (Make sure you only have one layer in your hand.) If the shirt has a seam, cut on the seam.

4. Lay the shirt either face up or down and take hold of the recently cut vertical line.

5. Turn the shirt so that the vertical line becomes a horizontal line from your perspective.

6. Cut slits (about 1 inch to 1 1/2 inches deep) down the side of the shirt, with about 1 inch to 3 inches between each incision.

7. Then lay the shirt so that the side with the incisions is facing up.

8. Tie each piece of fabric with the one across from it.

9. Slightly pull the fabric around each surrounding knot.

10. Flip to the other side and repeat steps 1–9.

Necklines (V and U)

WHAT YOU WILL NEED:

Flat surface to cut on

T-shirt

Ruler

Pencil

Scissors

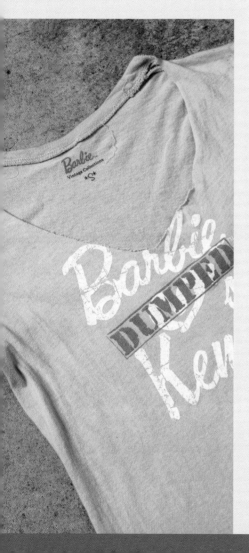

KEEP IN MIND: You can always take fabric away, but you can't add it.

WHAT TO DO:

1. On a flat surface, lay the T-shirt on its side with one of the shoulders facing up. (When you lay it like this, there should be a fold down the front and one down the back.)

2. For a V-neck, use a ruler and pencil and draw a slanted line on the neckline. The closer the line starts to the shoulder, the more plunging the neckline will be. (For U-necks, omit this step.)

3. Take the scissors and, starting from the point of the V, work your way up along the line. For a U-neck, start cutting where you want the lowest part of the U to be. Keep cutting a curved line until you reach the neckline.

4. Unfold the shirt and lay it down face up. Look to see whether you need any alterations. If so, fold the shirt on its side again and start cutting again, using the same technique as described in step 3, until you have the neckline you want.

Tube-Top Neckline

Difficulty: ★

WHAT YOU WILL NEED:

T-shirt

Flat surface to cut on

Ruler

Pencil

Scissors

KEEP IN MIND: You're making a tube top, so make sure the fabric won't slide down.

WHAT TO DO:

1. Lay the T-shirt face up on a flat surface.

2. Use a ruler and pencil to draw a straight, horizontal line from under one armpit to the other.

3. Take the scissors and cut across the line.

4. If the tube top is too big, you could always try adding knots to tighten the fit (see Knots Down the Sides on page 48 or Knots Down the Back on page 46 for instructions).

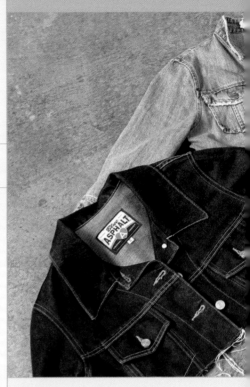

Mini Jean Jacket

Difficulty: ★

WHAT YOU WILL NEED:

Jean jacket

Flat surface to cut on

Ruler

Pencil

Scissors

Optional: needle and thread (or sewing machine) and pins

KEEP IN MIND: The jacket will not be as warm when you've shortened it; this is more of a fashion statement.

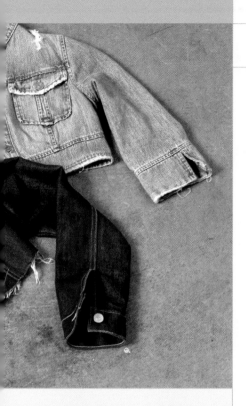

Ripped Jeans

WHAT YOU WILL NEED:

Jeans

Pencil

Flat surface to cut on

Scissors

Optional: cheese grater

KEEP IN MIND: Cut in places that would be naturally likely to have rips and holes.

WHAT TO DO:

1. Slip on the pair of jeans you want to cut up and mark with a pencil where you would like to have holes.

2. Place the jeans on a flat surface with the front facing up.

3. Use scissors to cut a tiny hole where you want there to be a rip.

4. Gently pull on the hole horizontally for a messy rip. The more you pull, the wider the rip will get.

5. Keep repeating steps 3 and 4 for all the rips you want to have.

6. Put the jeans in the washer and dryer, and they should come out having more fringe around the rips. The more you wear the jeans, the more fashionably ragged they will appear.

7. Optional: To make jeans look worn but not have rips and holes, you can use a cheese grater to make worn patches on the denim.

WHAT TO DO:

1. Choose a jean jacket (or any jacket for that matter) and lay it on a flat surface. You may want to button it first for accuracy.

2. Use your ruler and pencil and draw a horizontal line (starting about 2 inches below the armpit) across the jacket. Optional: If you want to sew the bottom of the jacket under for a cleaner line, measure 4 inches below the armpit instead of 2 inches.

3. With sissors, cut off the bottom of the jacket and any extra threads that are hanging.

4. Optional: To sew the bottom of the jacket under, fold the bottom layer under about 2 inches and pin it in place. Use either a needle and thread or sewing machine and sew around the bottom for a cleaner look.

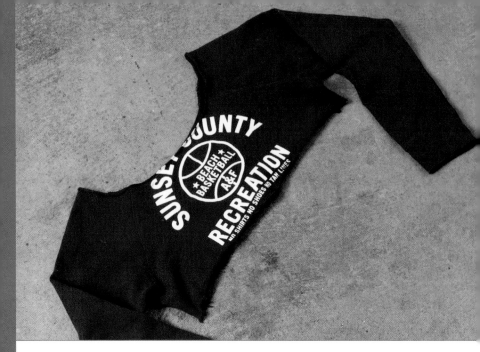

Cut Sweatshirt

Difficulty: ★

WHAT YOU WILL NEED:

Sweatshirt

Flat surface to cut on

Ruler

Pencil

Scissors

KEEP IN MIND: Using a slimmer-fitting sweatshirt will look better.

WHAT TO DO:

1. Lay the sweatshirt face up on a flat surface.

2. With the ruler and pencil, mark a point on either side about 2 inches away from the shoulder.

3. Draw a curving line that connects both points.

4. Before cutting out the neckline, move to the bottom of the sweatshirt.

5. Depending on how long you want the sweatshirt to be, use your ruler and pencil and draw a straight line across the sweatshirt.

6. Use your scissors and cut out the neckline, making sure you cut out the back at the same time.

7. Cut the bottom of the sweatshirt. Start out cutting a little lower than you think best, because you can always take fabric away, but you can't add it.

8. Try it on and look to see whether you want to make any alterations. If not, wear it, girl!

Suggestion for wearing: You could wear the sweatshirt off one shoulder with the sleeves rolled up, or you could wear it off both shoulders.

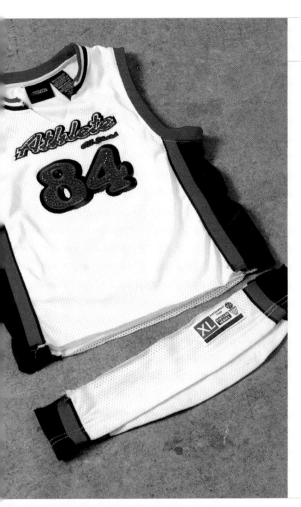

Jersey Belt

Difficulty: ★

WHAT YOU WILL NEED:

Fitted jersey

Flat surface to cut on

Ruler

Pencil

Scissors

Optional: needle and thread
(or sewing machine)

KEEP IN MIND: You can purchase an inexpensive fitted jersey from the little boys' section of most department stores.

WHAT TO DO:

1. Lay the jersey on a flat surface.

2. Use a ruler and pencil to draw a horizontal line across the bottom of the jersey. The jersey belt should be at least 3 inches thick.

3. Use scissors to cut along the horizontal line.

4. Optional: To preserve your jersey belt, use a needle and thread (or sewing machine, if you can operate one) to sew the rough edge down.

Suggestion for wearing: It's hot to wear the jersey belt you make with the jersey that it came from (see page 69).

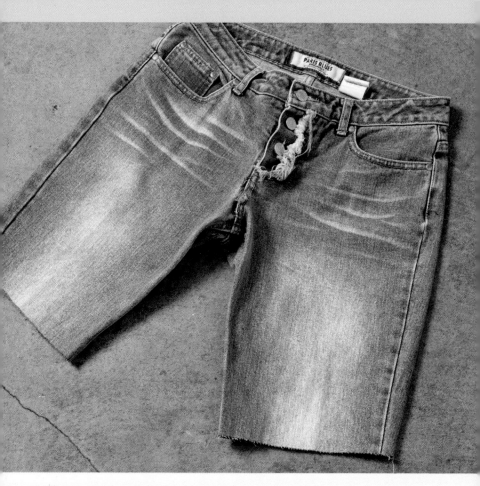

Short Jean Pants

Difficulty: ★

WHAT YOU WILL NEED:

Jeans

Pencil

Flat surface to cut on

Ruler

Scissors

KEEP IN MIND: Jeans that are a little baggier will work better than fitted jeans.

WHAT TO DO:

1. Try the jeans on that you are about to make into short pants.

2. With a pencil, draw a line right above one knee.

3. Take the jeans off and lay them on a flat surface.

4. Use a ruler and pencil to draw a straight line across where you marked in the previous step.

5. Use scissors to cut across the line.

6. Repeat for the other leg.

Fingerless Gloves

Difficulty: ★

WHAT YOU WILL NEED:

Gloves

Pencil

Flat surface to cut on

Ruler

Scissors

KEEP IN MIND: Only thin gloves work for this.

WHAT TO DO:

1. Put on the first glove that you would like to cut up.

2. Use a pencil to make a straight line where you want the cut to be, starting at your pinky and going all the way across to your pointer finger. Make sure that the horizontal line is below the middle joint in your ring, middle, and pointer fingers.

3. Place the glove on a flat surface. Use a ruler and pencil to draw a straight line across where you marked in the previous step.

4. Take your scissors and cut across the lines made in steps 2 and 3.

5. Put the glove on and make any adjustments.

6. Make a line, using the pencil, below your wrist bone.

7. Take the glove off and cut along the line.

8. Repeat for the other glove, and you're done!

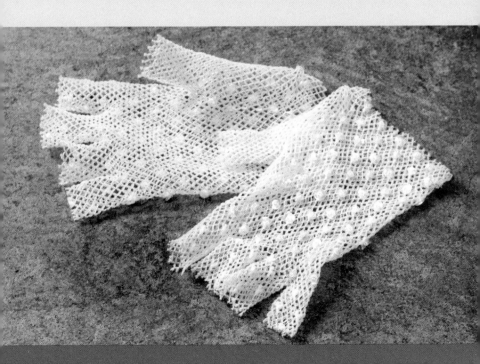

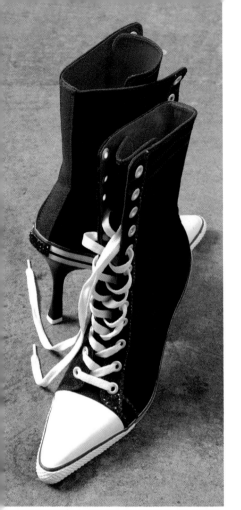

THE ART OF CRYSTALS

When it comes to crystalling things, it's all about creativity. There is one way to crystal things, and this same technique applies to anything you want to do: You always start with a line (vertical or horizontal). If you are going to crystal an entire design, first crystal the outline and work your way into the center in a circular motion (clockwise or counterclockwise, it doesn't really matter, whatever's easiest for you). You can apply this technique to crystalling shirts, pants, jerseys, cell phones, purses, skirts, shoes, etc.

Keep in mind that the more crystals you use, the higher the price of the project. You'd better be sure from the beginning that you want to sink the money, as well as the time, into whatever project you're thinking about. It's very rare to use only one gross of crystals (144); usually, I use three, four, or even six gross for a project!

There are many different sizes of crystals, including 5ss, 7ss, 9ss, 12ss, 16ss, 20ss, 30ss, 34ss, 40ss, 42ss, and 48ss. The larger the number, the bigger the crystal. (Just to give you an idea of size, 48ss is about the size of a nickel, 30ss is the size of a penny, and 5ss is a little bigger than the head of a pin.) The price range for one gross of 5ss is $5.49, of 16ss it's $6.99, and of 48ss it's $98! I personally have never used crystals larger than 20ss, because the smaller the crystals, the more bling-bling. Before you buy, determine what size would be best to use for the project you are going to work on. Keep in mind that if you are a beginner, it's best to start out using crystal sizes 16ss and 20ss. It's harder to manipulate smaller crystals.

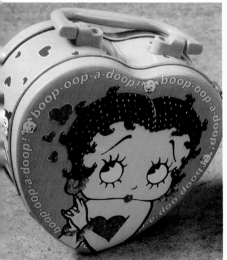

Crystal Sunglasses

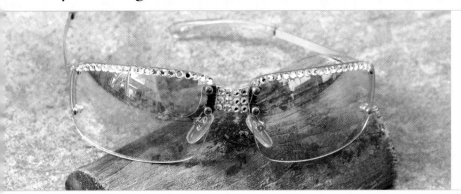

Difficulty: ★★★

WHAT YOU WILL NEED:

Either Austrian or
Swarovski crystals
(amount differs)

Flat surface to work on

Different colors of
construction paper

Flat dish for crystals

Toothpicks

E6000 glue

Paper towels

Sunglasses

KEEP IN MIND: Sunglasses without
frames are best.

WHAT TO DO:

1. Purchase about two gross of crystals in whatever color you want.
   (One gross contains 144 crystals.)
   You should get about size 12ss or
   smaller (but remember, the smaller
   the crystal size, the harder they
   are to apply).

2. Set up a "crystal station" on a flat
   surface. Lay down a piece of construction paper that is a different
   color than the crystals you're
   using. You should also have a dish
   with some crystals sparkly side up.

Have a few toothpicks ready and a
"safe" place to have E6000 glue drip
(paper towel recommended!).

3. Have sunglass lenses facing up for
   easier work.

4. Using a toothpick, get a small
   amount of glue and make a line
   at the top of the lenses.

5. Using the toothpick, with only a
   miniscule amount of glue on it, pick
   up crystals one by one and put them
   on the glue line on the glasses.

6. Keep repeating until you get the
   desired look.

7. To crystal the sides of the sunglasses,
   open one of the arms (leave the other
   one folded in).

8. If there is a design, take a toothpick
   and get some E6000 glue on it.
   Trace the design with the glue and
   stick crystals on (be quick—the glue
   sets fast). If there isn't a design,
   crystal about half of the arm. Use a
   toothpick to make horizontal lines
   and place crystals on them.

9. Repeat until you're done.

10. Wait about 30 minutes to an hour
    before wearing.

CONVERSIONS

In this section, I will show you how to convert different things into something more fashionable or more useful, or a combination of the two!

Converting Pierced Earrings to Clip-Ons

Difficulty: ★

WHAT YOU WILL NEED:

Pair of pierced earrings

Pliers

Clip-on earring backs

WHAT TO DO:

1. Choose a pair of earrings that you would like to make into clip-ons. Pretty much any earring will do except hoops and studs.

2. Locate a loop at the top of the earring that connects the stud to the dangling part.

3. Use your pliers to open (separate) the loop that is at the bottom of the stud and is holding the dangling part of the earring.

4. Hold the dangling earring by the loop that was connected to the stud in the previous step.

5. Slide the loop inside the open loop of the clip-on earring.

6. Use the pliers to shut the loop of the clip-on.

7. Repeat for the other earring.

8. Ta da! You're done, and they are ready to wear.

9. Optional: If the clip-on is too tight, you can use the pliers to squeeze the back of the earring farther away from the front to make the gap bigger. If the clip-on is too loose, you can use your pliers to pull the earring back closer to the earring front so that the gap is smaller.

Jean Purse

Difficulty: ★★

WHAT YOU WILL NEED:

Jeans

Flat surface to cut on

Ruler

Pencil

Scissors

Straight pins

Needle and thread
(or sewing machine)

Screwdriver

Optional: silver O-rings and pins, buttons, broaches, or safety pins for decoration

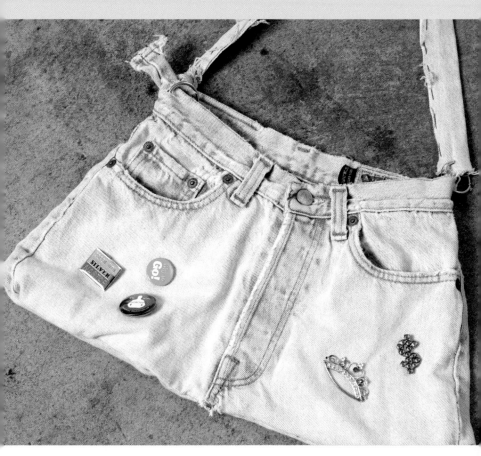

WHAT TO DO:

1. Take a pair of jeans that you want to make into a purse and lay them on a flat surface.

2. Use your ruler and pencil to draw a horizontal line slightly above the crotch.

3. Use your scissors to cut across the horizontal line.

4. With your ruler and pencil, draw two parallel vertical lines (about 2 inches apart) along one of the cut-off leg scraps.

5. Cut the strip out and put it aside for later use.

6. Turn the denim (which now looks like a skirt) inside out. Use straight pins to pin along the open bottom end of the purse.

7. Take a needle and thread (or sewing machine, if you can operate one) and sew along the pinned edge.

8. Turn the bag right side out and look to see whether you need to make any alterations.

9. Take the strip of denim from step 5 and sew along the edge to make a purse shoulder strap.

10. Either sew the shoulder strap on or punch a hole (using a screw-driver) through both sides of the bag and both ends of the shoulder strap and connect using two silver O-rings.

11. Optional: Add pins, buttons, brooches, or safety pins as decorations.

Bleach Stains

Difficulty: ★

WHAT YOU WILL NEED:

Denim jeans, skirt, shorts, etc.

Bleach

Spray bottle

Rubber gloves

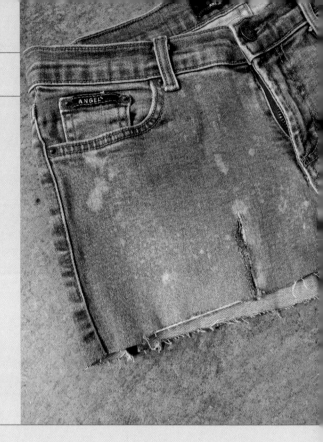

WHAT TO DO:

1. Lay the denim that you want to bleach in a bathtub or sink (whichever is more convenient).

2. Pour a small amount of bleach into a spray bottle. (Warning: Once you use a spray bottle for bleach, that is all it should be used for from there on out.)

3. Put on rubber gloves. Spray the denim with bleach from about 2 feet away for a more speckled look. For a blotchier look, spray at a closer range, but always maintain at least a 6-inch distance between the spray bottle and the denim.

4. Spray a little bleach into your rubber-gloved hand and gently massage the bleach into the denim in different locations.

5. Let the bleach set, and you should see the results when the denim is dry.

Patch Jacket

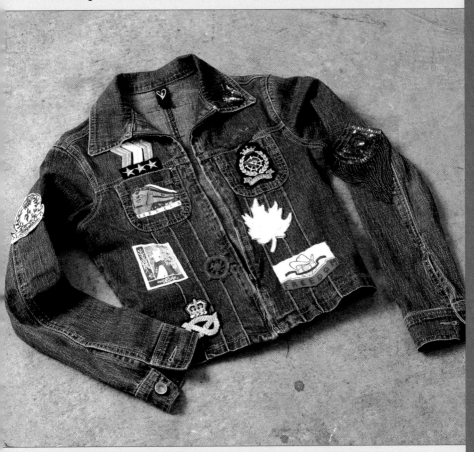

Difficulty: ★★

WHAT YOU WILL NEED:

Jacket

Flat surface to work on

An array of different patches
(or fabric swatches)

Straight pins

Needle and thread (or
sewing machine)

WHAT TO DO:

1. Lay the jacket on a flat surface.

2. Place the patches where you want
   them to be on the jacket and
   secure them with straight pins.

3. Use either a needle and thread or a
   sewing machine (if you can operate
   one) to sew on the patches.

4. Wear it!

Toothbrush Bracelet

Difficulty: ★★

WHAT YOU WILL NEED:

Plastic toothbrush

2 pairs of pliers

Cooking pot

WHAT TO DO:

1. Pull the toothbrush bristles out with a pair of pliers.

2. Boil the toothbrush in a pot of water on the stove until it can be shaped.

3. Use the two pairs of pliers to bend the brush into a circular shape. (Leave about 1/4 of an inch between the ends of the toothbrush.)

4. Let the toothbrush bracelet cool.

Switching Buttons

Difficulty: ★★

WHAT YOU WILL NEED:

Buttons (the number should match how many buttons are on the garment already)

Garment

Scissors

Needle and thread

Optional: E6000 glue and crystals

WHAT TO DO:

1. Choose buttons that you would like to put on the garment.

2. Use the scissors to remove the original buttons.

3. Sew on the new buttons with needle and thread.

4. Ta da! You're done.

5. Suggestion: If the original buttons can't be removed, try gluing crystals over them, or just glue one gigantic crystal on top of each button (see The Art of Crystals on page 56 for how to choose and apply crystals).

OTHER CRAFTY CREATIONS

Finally, I'd like to include a few miscellaneous projects that don't really fit anywhere else. But I love them anyway!

Painted Cowboy Hat

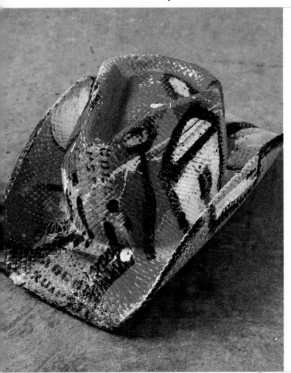

Difficulty: ★★

WHAT YOU WILL NEED:

Newspaper or cardboard

Cowboy hat

Fabric or acrylic paint

Paper towels

Paintbrushes

KEEP IN MIND: You can also use this technique to paint shoes, skirts, pants, purses; you name it. The sky's the limit!

WHAT TO DO:

1. Set up your painting station: Place newspaper or cardboard underneath the cowboy hat and have a palette of paint colors (don't be afraid to mix them), water, paper towels, and paintbrushes nearby.

2. Be creative and just start painting away! Don't forget to wash your brush out before you use the next color.

3. Let the cowboy hat dry overnight.

HOT TIP

A wet brush won't make the colors show up as vibrantly on the cowboy hat, so dry off your brush after every dip in water.

Tie-Dyeing

WHAT YOU WILL NEED:

T-shirt, skirt, or other garment

Rubber bands

Food coloring

Plastic bowl

Rubber gloves

Optional: crystals

WHAT TO DO:

1. Choose a garment that you would like to tie-dye. Scrunch it into a ball and tie it several times with rubber bands.

2. Choose a food color to tie-dye the garment with, keeping in mind that the color won't be as vibrant as it looks in the bottle. (I use food coloring right out of our kitchen. If you would like to use real fabric dye, remember that it is more expensive.)

3. Fill a plastic bowl with water. Put many drops of food coloring in until the water is a solid color (mix with a utensil, if needed).

4. Put on rubber gloves and place the garment in the bowl. Keep submerging it for a darker color.

5. Squeeze the garment dry to get excess water out and put drops of food coloring on the garment. Massage the color in with your rubber glove.

6. Keep repeating steps 4 and 5 until you get the desired look.

7. Take the rubber bands off and let the garment air-dry on a drying rack (mentioned on page 32).

8. Optional: Add crystals when the garment is dry (see The Art of Crystals on page 56).

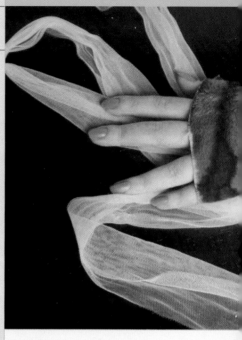

Tiger Armband

Difficulty: ★

WHAT YOU WILL NEED:

Scissors

Fabric (get about 1/2 yard so you have room to mess up)

Straight pins

Needle and thread (or sewing machine)

Optional: pins and patches

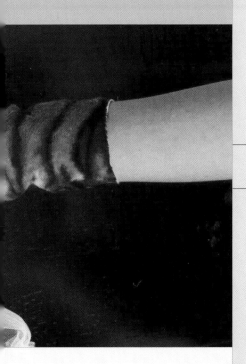

Button Necklace

Difficulty: ★

WHAT YOU WILL NEED:

Wire cutters

Wire (about 1 foot)

Buttons

Beads (no more than 10)

Clasp

WHAT TO DO:

1. Using wire cutters, cut a long piece of wire (about 1 foot). Make an O at one end and wrap some of the wire around it so that the buttons and beads won't fall off.

2. Start putting buttons on. Use all different sizes and add beads periodically.

3. Once you've made the necklace as long as you want, make an O at the other end and wrap the excess wire around.

4. Attach the clasp to the necklace and wear.

WHAT TO DO:

1. Use scissors to cut the fabric so that the length is about 5 1/2 inches.

2. Cut the fabric so that the width is around 7 inches (give or take some, depending on how small or big your wrist is).

3. Pin along the edges of the fabric to make a loop. Make sure that you're pinning so that the seam will be on the inside.

4. Either with a needle and thread or a sewing machine, stitch the edges together. Leave about a 1/2 inch at each end so that there is room to put your hand in.

5. Remove the straight pins and wear!

6. Optional: Add pins and patches.

7. The Ensembles

The pages about to unfold in front of you show the outfits I styled to help you create the wardrobe you've always wanted. You may notice that I did not use professional models for this book. They are all real girls with real, healthy figures. I wanted to show that you don't have to be a stick figure to look good. Matter of fact, these girls are all high school students and my friends.

If you are going to wear a fedora, make sure you're wearing it slightly to the side. Pull it down a bit to give off a mysterious vibe.

FAIRY PRINCESS

HAT: Miguel Torres
NECKLACE: Lee Riot
UNDERSHIRT: Rojas
TUBE TOP: Forever 21
BRACELET: Marciano
RING: Chinatown in New York City
BELT: Ecko Red
SKIRT: Hot Kiss
HEELS: Michael Antonio

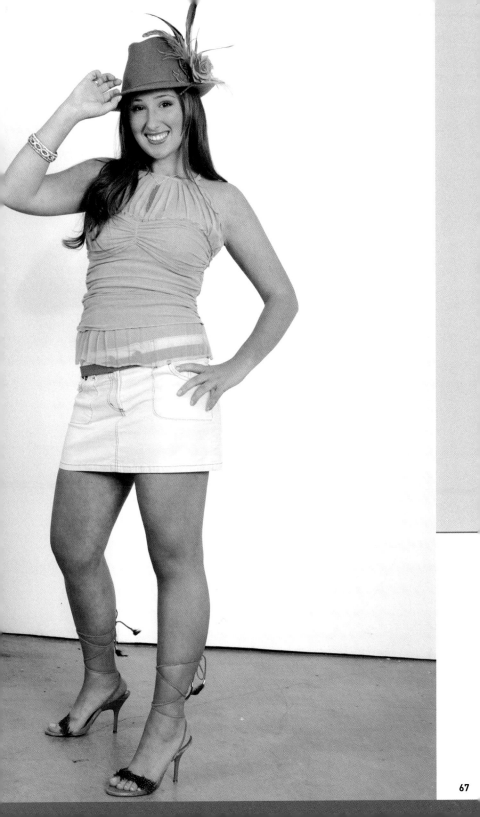

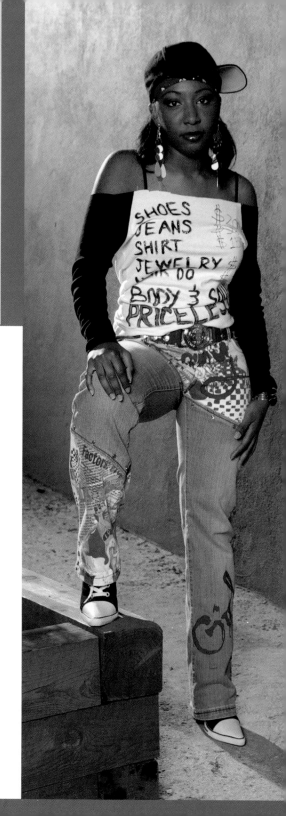

A classic color combination—black, red, and white. Remember to have fun with them, and when you put an outfit together using those classics make sure you wear accessories that are the same three colors.

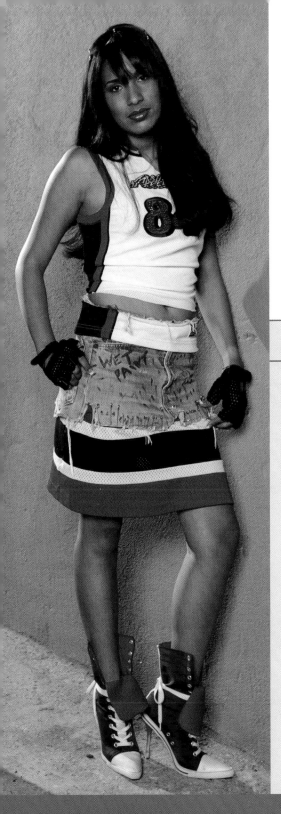

URBAN

RACING FLAG (left)

BASEBALL HAT: garment district of Los Angeles
BANDANA: EOEO
EARRINGS: Rampage
TOP: Amber's Escapades
BRACELET: Marianna's Designer Jewelry
BELT: Ecko Red
PANTS: Johnny Girl
HEELS: Steve Madden

AMERICANA (right)

SUNGLASSES: garment district of Los Angeles
TOP: personal creation
WORKOUT GLOVES: Bello
BELT: personal creation
SKIRT: Amber's Escapades
HEELS: Steve Madden

I like these three outfits together because they complement each other and have the same flavor.

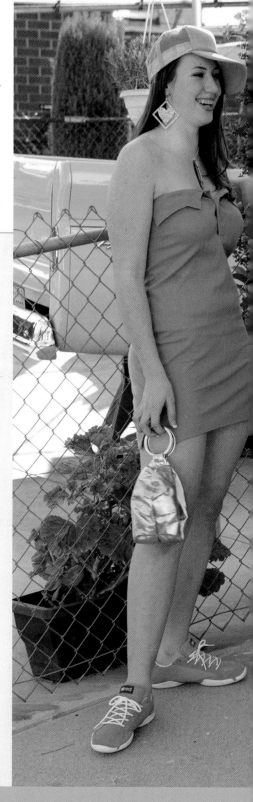

BLUE RIBBON (left)

TRUCKER HAT: Rock & Republic
EARRINGS: Lee Riot
NECKLACE: Lee Riot
DRESS: Rojas
BRACELET: Lee Riot
HANDBAG: inexpensive boutique
TENNIS SHOES: Ecko Red

GI JANE (center)

EARRINGS: Amber's Escapades
NECKLACES: Lee Riot
DRESS: G Unit
BRACELET: Kenneth Cole
BELT: Leatherock
HEELS: Ecko Red

SCHOOL BOY (right)

BEANIE: Bonknits by Bonnie
EARRINGS: Lee Riot
NECKLACE: Lee Riot
TOP: Rojas
BRACELET: Cheyne Hauk
MESSENGER BAG: New York City Subway Line
BELT: Leatherock
PANTS: G Unit
TENNIS SHOES: Converse

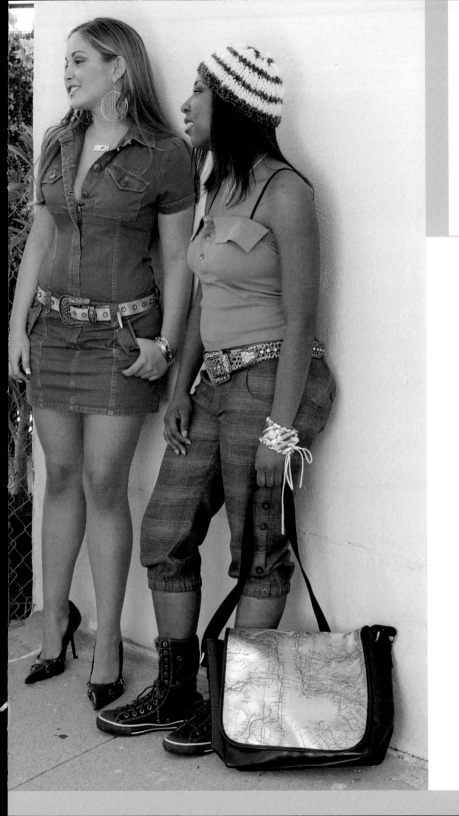

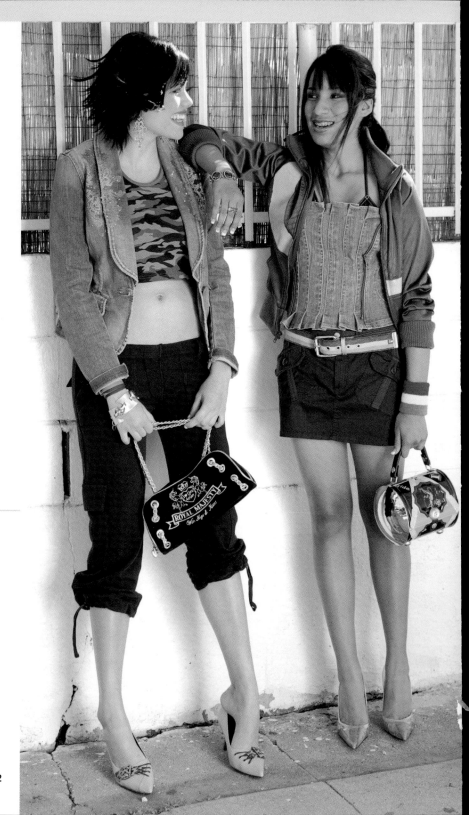

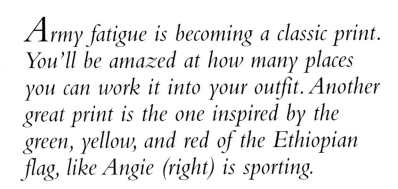

Army fatigue is becoming a classic print. You'll be amazed at how many places you can work it into your outfit. Another great print is the one inspired by the green, yellow, and red of the Ethiopian flag, like Angie (right) is sporting.

SERPENT (left)

EARRINGS: Kenneth Cole

BLAZER: Marciano

TOP: Johnny Girl

BRACELET: Marianna's Designer Jewelry

SWEATPANTS: Bebe

HANDBAG: Wal-Mart

HEELS: Michael Antonio

ETHIOPIA (right)

JACKET: Catch A Fire

BIKINI TOP: Akademiks

TUBE TOP: Akademiks

BRACELET: Marianna's Designer Jewelry

WRISTBAND: Claire's

RING: Amber's Escapades

BELT: Ecko Red

SKIRT: Triple 5 Soul

HANDBAG: Little Earth

HEELS: Steve Madden

I love the color turquoise. It looks good on every skin tone. Coral, lavender, hot pink, oranges, olive green, and your basic black, white, and gray are all great complements to turquoise.

CHLORINE (left)

NECKLACE: Lee Riot
ZIP-UP HOODIE: Miken
JACKET: Miken
BRACELET: Amber's Escapades
SEQUINED GLOVES: personal creation
BELT: Ecko Red
SWEATPANTS: Akademiks
TENNIS SHOES: Ecko Red

AQUAMARINE (right)

EARRINGS: Marianna's Designer Jewelry
TOP: Akademiks
BELT: Ecko Red
PANTS: Akademiks
WORKOUT GLOVES: Bello
HEELS: Ecko Red

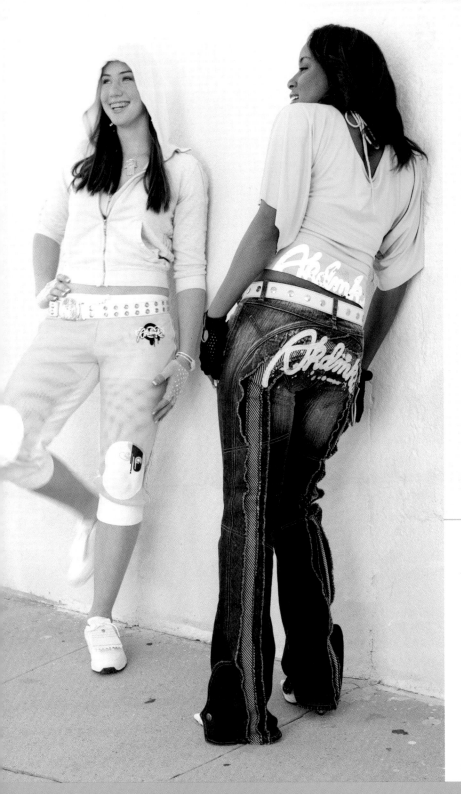

I don't actually expect anyone to walk around with a big furry hood on her head and a dress; this was just for show. As far as kneesocks and wristbands go, though, those are always great accessories to add instead of going with the standard jewelry.

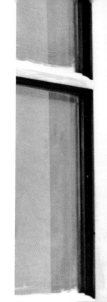

ESKIMO (left)

HOOD: Rocawear
TUBE TOP: Forever 21
DRESS: Rojas
BRACELET: Cheyne Hauk
BRACELET AND RING: Marianna's Designer Jewelry
BELT: Leatherock
LEG WARMERS: Adidas
HEELS: Roach Killers

WARPED (right)

TRUCKER HAT: Beverly Hills Pimps & Ho's
EARRINGS: Amber's Escapades
JACKET: Rojas
TOP: Akademiks
WRISTBAND: Von Dutch
BRACELET: Marianna's Designer Jewelry
BELT: Ecko Red
SKIRT: Rojas
HEELS: Michael Antonio

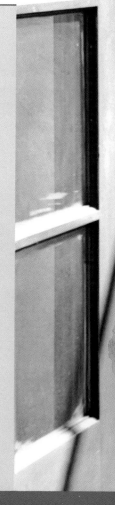

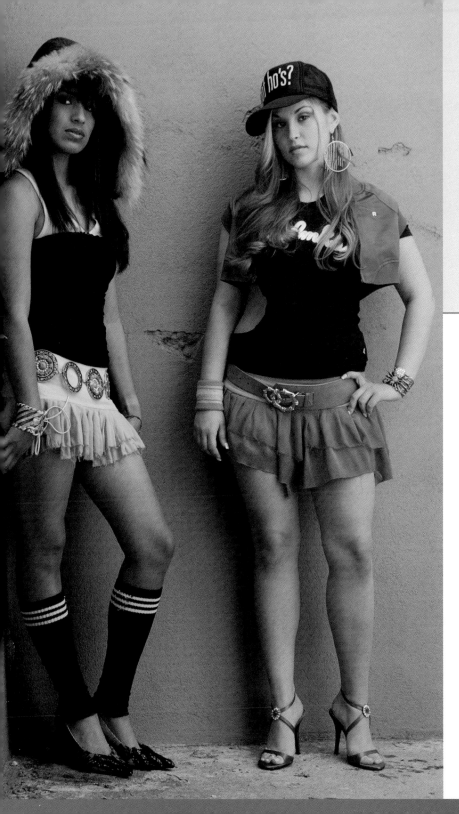

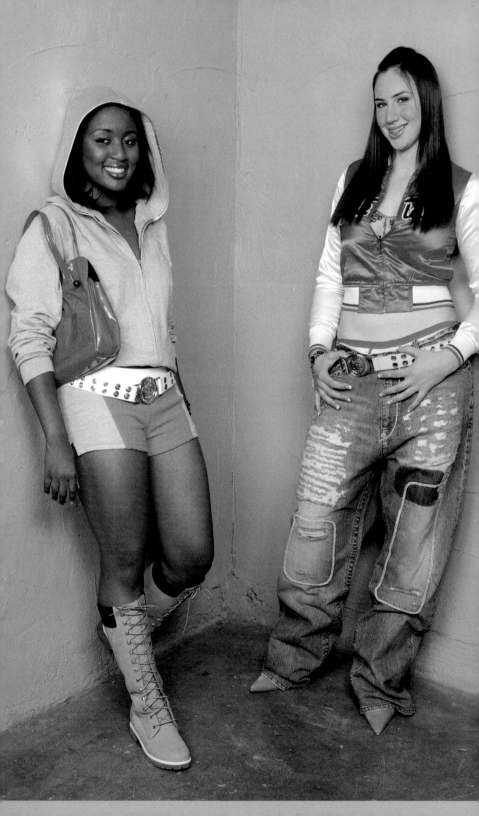

Sometimes it's fun to dress a little bit more on the tomboy side gone glam. If you do, make sure you add in some feminine pieces as well as some jewelry.

URBAN CONSTRUCTION (left)

JACKET: Rojas
PURSE: vintage
BELT: Ecko Red
SHORTS: Miken
BOOTS: Timberland

HOODWINK (right)

JACKET: Blue Marlin
BRA: Marianna's Designer Jewelry
BOY PANTIES: Windsor
BELT: Ecko Red
BRACELET: Marianna's Designer Jewelry
DENIM JEANS [MEN'S]: Akademiks
BOOTS: Michael Antonio

I like to throw in a bright element here and there when dealing with a predominantly dark outfit.

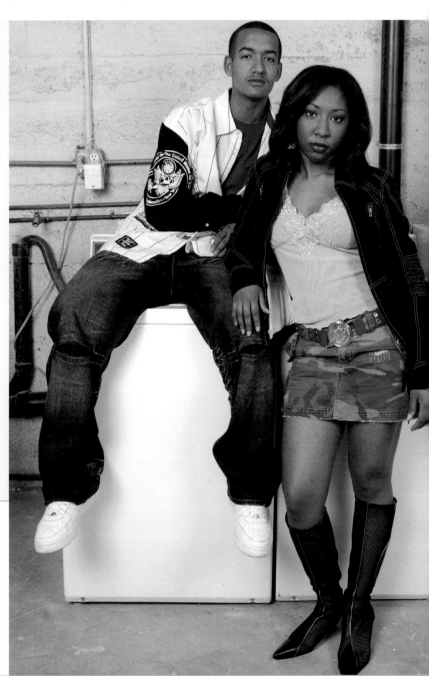

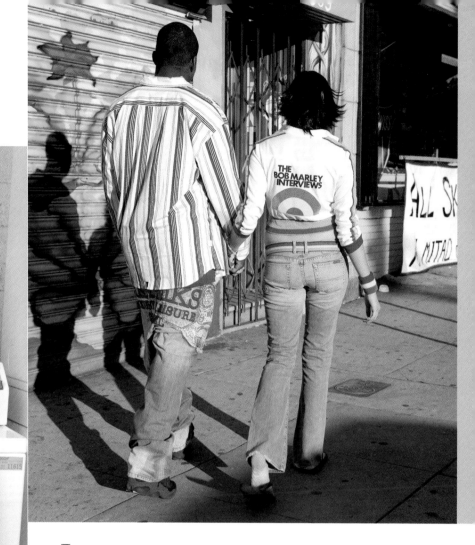

I think it's awesome when most of
the detail is on the back of the outfit.

RAVAGE (left)

JACKET: Akademiks
TOP: Forever 21
BELT: Ecko Red
SKIRT: Ecko Red
BOOTS: Michael Antonio

SOMEWHERE ELSE (above)

JACKET: Catch A Fire
BRACELET: Lee Riot
WRISTBAND: Claire's
BELT: Ecko Red
DENIM JEANS: Lucky Brand Jeans
SANDALS: Old Navy

*W*hat I like about these outfits is that they are chill, but they are still fashionable at the same time. The key to a "chill" look is wearing comfy, casual clothes and throwing in a fashion flare with a jacket, hat, belt, and jewelry.

GLACE AU CAFÉ (left)

CAP: Peter Grimm Headwear

HEART NECKLACE: Marianna's Designer Jewelery

FEATHER NECKLACE: inexpensive boutique

TURQUOISE NECKLACE: Rampage

TANK: inexpensive boutique

JACKET: Rojas

HANDBAG: Fetish

WRISTBAND: Claire's

BELT: Ecko Red

DENIM JEANS: Hot Kiss

TENNIS SHOES: Converse

CARBONATED (right)

CAP: Peter Grimm Headwear

EARRINGS: Urban Outfitters

ZIP-UP JACKET: Roxy

BOMBER JACKET: Abercrombie & Fitch

T-SHIRT: Junk Food

NECKLACE: personal creation

CLUTCH: Your Sister's Mustache

BELT: Little Earth

DENIM JEANS: Lucky Brand Jeans

TENNIS SHOES: Converse

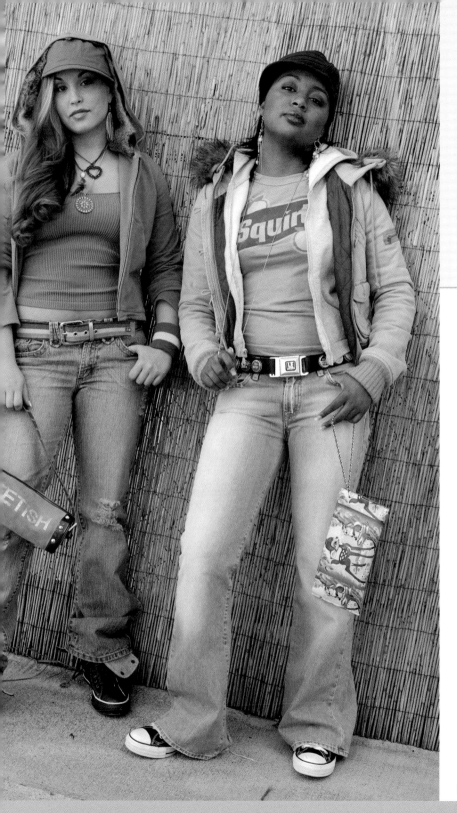

*T*hese outfits would typically be worn to either a club or a concert. When you put an outfit together to go out, of course, you want to be a little showy and risqué. It's definitely okay to go all out and dress like some music video girls, if you can pull it off.

CAFFEINE (left)

HAT: Beverly Hills Pimps & Ho's
FLOWER: Sleaze
EARRINGS: Marianna's Designer Jewelry
TUBE TOP: inexpensive boutique
HANDBAG: Fetish
BRACELET: vintage
BELT: Fetish
KEY CHAIN: Bebe
SKIRT: Forever 21
HEELS: Charlotte Russe

ENVY (right)

EARRINGS: Claire's
TANK: inexpensive boutique
BRACELET: Kenneth Cole
HANDBAG: Fetish
BELT: Ecko Red
SWEATPANTS: Bebe
BOOTS: Michael Antonio

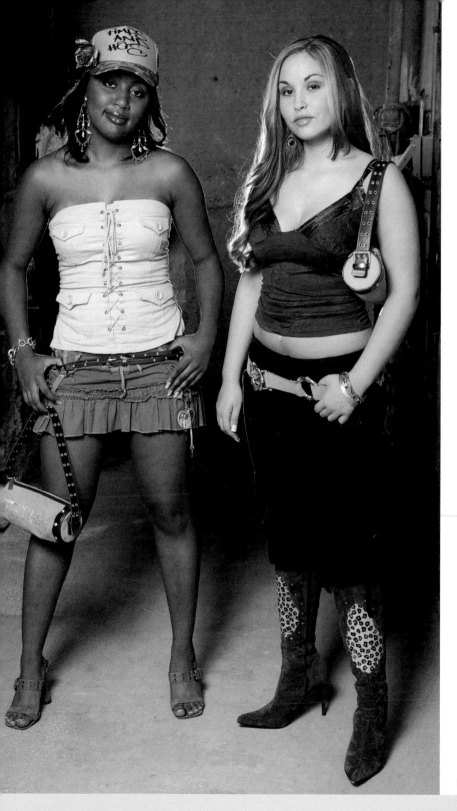

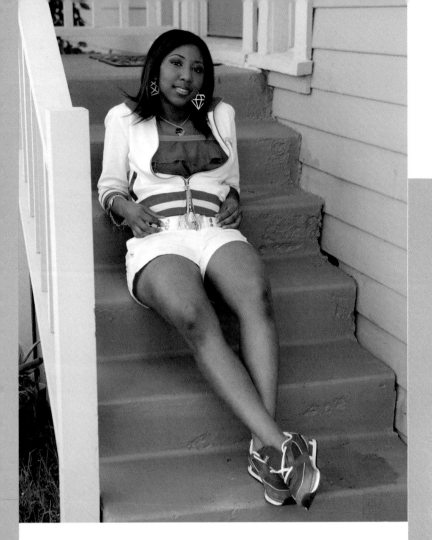

Wearing a matching jacket really does pull a look together.

PURPLE CRUSH (above)

EARRINGS: Lee Riot
NECKLACE: Lee Riot
JACKET: Rocawear
TOP: Rojas
BRACELET: Lee Riot
BELT: Ecko Red
SHORTS: Roxy
TENNIS SHOES: Ecko Red

BRIGHT AUTUMN (right)

NECKLACES: Lee Riot
TOP: Custo
BOMBER JACKET: Triple 5 Soul
BELT: Leatherock
SWEATPANTS: personal creation
BOOTS: Michael Antonio

Cutting off baggy sweatpants at the knee gives off the impression of Bermuda shorts or a knee-length skirt, and can be dressed up or down. These long shorts work with every body type, unless you have thick calves.

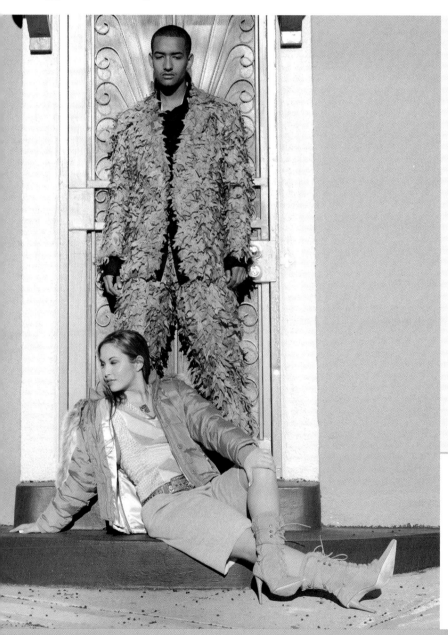

I put these outfits together because they both have a little bit of the same color scheme, but they come off as two really different looks. Long, dangling jewelry is the best. It always makes a vertical statement, creating length and height. Wearing long earrings or necklaces also takes the burden away from accessorizing further. (Although, that is still an option.)

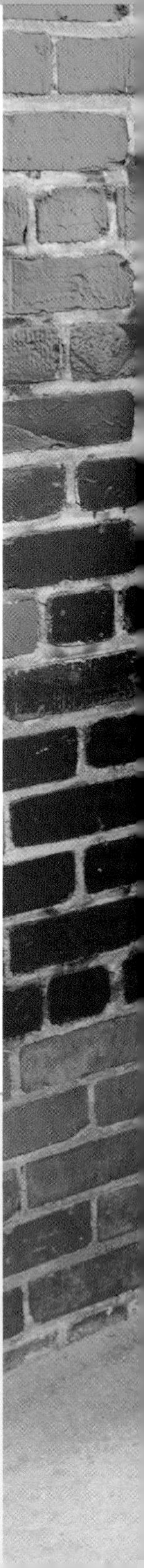

PASSION FRUIT (left)

NECKLACE AND BELLY CHAIN:
Marianna's Designer Jewelry

PEARLS: Rite Aid

SWEATSHIRT: G Unit

BRACELET: Marciano

HANDBAG: Baby Phat

SKIRT: Hot Kiss

HEELS: Michael Antonio

HUMID RASPBERRY
(right)

EARRINGS: Rampage

BOMBER JACKET: Abercrombie
& Fitch

SHIRT: Miken

SWEATPANTS: Miken

HANDBAG: Marciano

HEELS: Michael Antonio

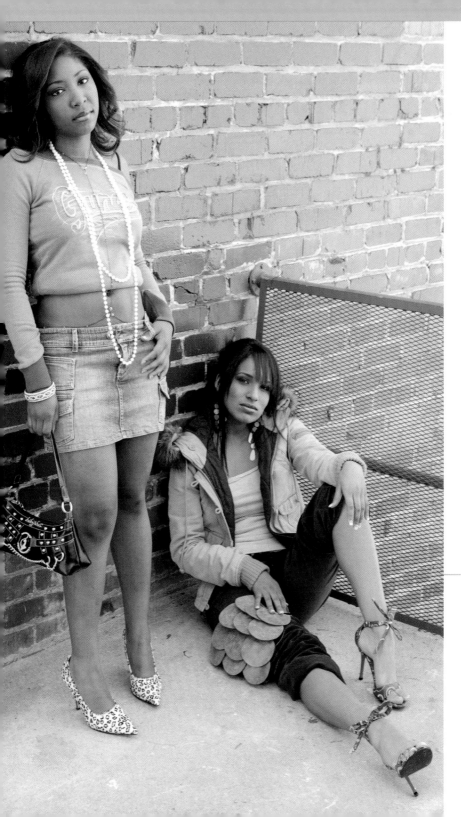

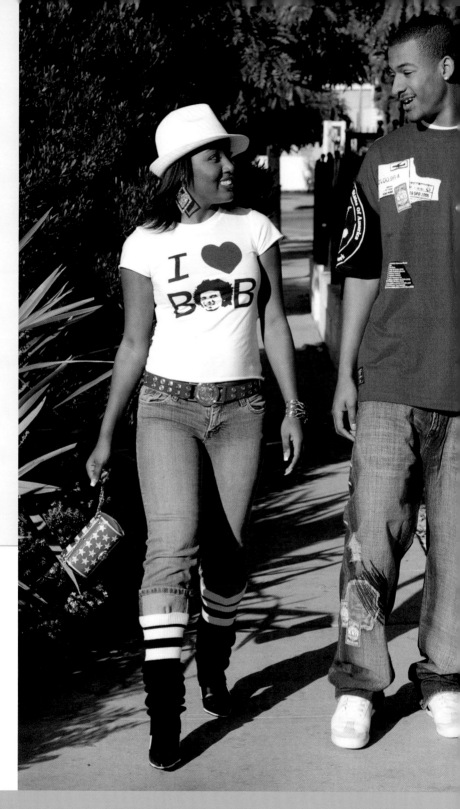

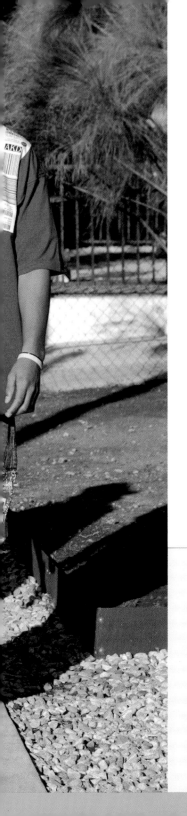

*W*hen having trouble coming up with an outfit, throw on a T-shirt and jeans and glam it up with some accessories. Make sure that your T-shirt is always untucked.

BOB

FEDORA: Peter Grimm Headwear

EARRINGS: Lee Riot

TOP: Catch A Fire

BRACELET: Marianna's Designer Jewelry

HANDBAG: Little Earth

BELT: Ecko Red

DENIM JEANS: Forever 21

BOOTS: Ecko Red

*T*urning belt buckles to the side widens your hips, making your body appear more hourglass-shaped.

DERELICT (left)

HEART NECKLACE: Sleaze

NECKLACE: vintage

JACKET: Target

MULTI-BRACELET: Kenneth Cole

HANDBAG: Your Sister's Mustache

BELT: Wal-Mart

DENIM JEANS: Lucky Brand Jeans

HEELS: Steve Madden

EAST COAST (right)

EARRINGS: Kenneth Cole

JACKET: Johnny Girl

NECKLACE AND BELLY CHAIN: Marianna's Designer Jewelry

SHIRT: personal creation

BRACELET: Lee Riot

DENIM JEANS: Lucky Brand Jeans

BOOTS: Michael Antonio

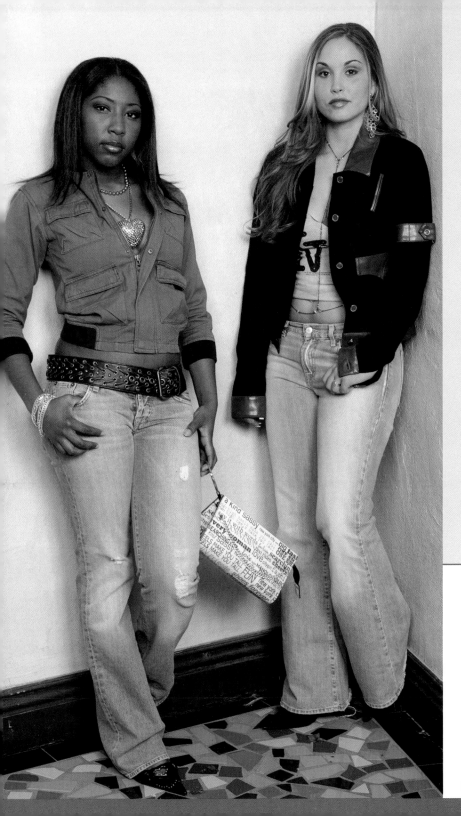

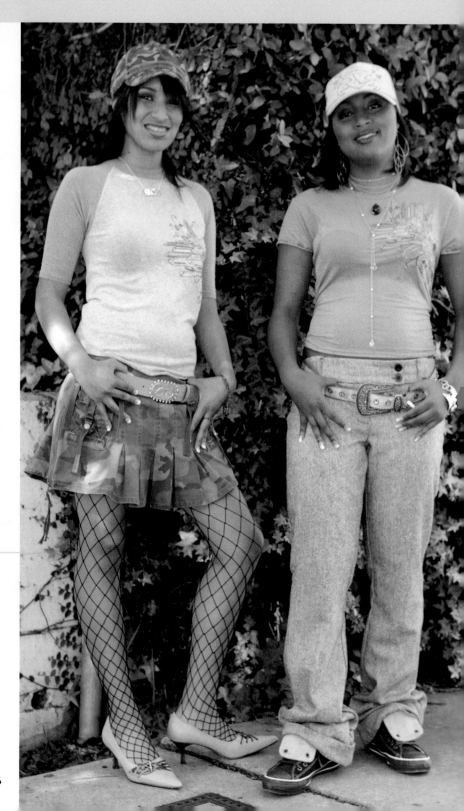

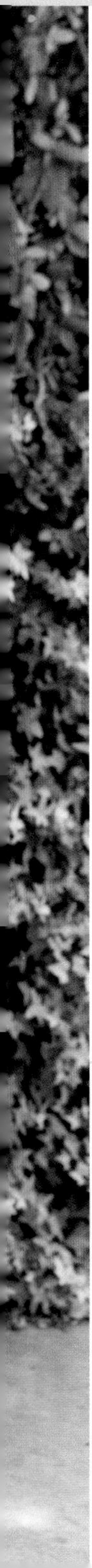

*P*laying around with different types of bottoms besides denim will usually make an outfit more interesting. Try playing around with velour, cotton, linen, etc. Also, experimenting with patterns like fatigue, tweed, and Asian-inspired designs, etc. can add another dimension to an otherwise plain outfit.

GEM (left)

HAT: Peter Grimm Headwear

NECKLACE: Lee Riot

SHIRT: Rojas

BRACELET: Marianna's Designer Jewelry

BELT: Ecko Red

SKIRT: Forever 21

FISHNETS: dance shop

HEELS: Michael Antonio

NACHO CHEESE (right)

TRUCKER HAT: H&M

EARRINGS: Gorjana

NECKLACES: Gorjana

TOP: Rojas

BRA: Chinese Laundry

BRACELET: Marianna's Designer Jewelry

BELT: Leatherock

PANTS: Forever 21

TENNIS SHOES: Converse

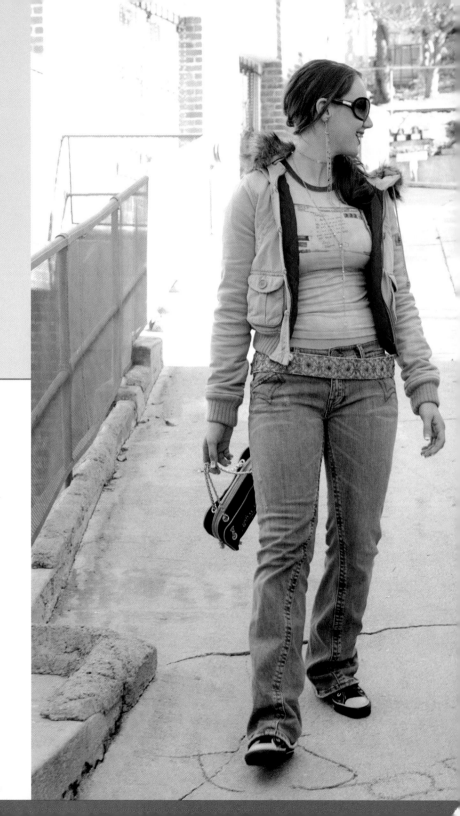

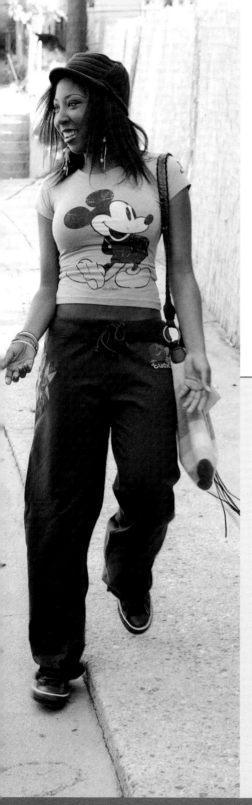

*Y*ou don't have to dress over the top every day! Some days it's best to stick with being casual. If you choose to go casual, avoid wearing crystals, sequins, or anything else super-flashy—it just doesn't look right.

INCOGNITO (left)

SUNGLASSES: drugstore
EARRINGS: Urban Outfitters
BOMBER JACKET: Abercrombie & Fitch
T-SHIRT: Dear John
NECKLACE: Gorjana
BELT: vintage
DENIM JEANS: Miss Me
HANDBAG: Wal-Mart
TENNIS SHOES: Converse

CHOCOLATE SPRINKLES
(right)

CAP: Peter Grimm Headwear
EARRINGS: Urban Outfitters
T-SHIRT: Vintage Peanuts
BRACELETS: inexpensive
Indian boutique
PURSE: Gap
SWEATPANTS: Lucky Brand Jeans
TENNIS SHOES: Converse

Generally speaking, flats with capris will visually shorten your legs. That is, unless you have extremely long, thin legs. Baseball shirts, like the one Jackie (left) is wearing, can be purchased at most sporting goods stores if you can't afford a designer one.

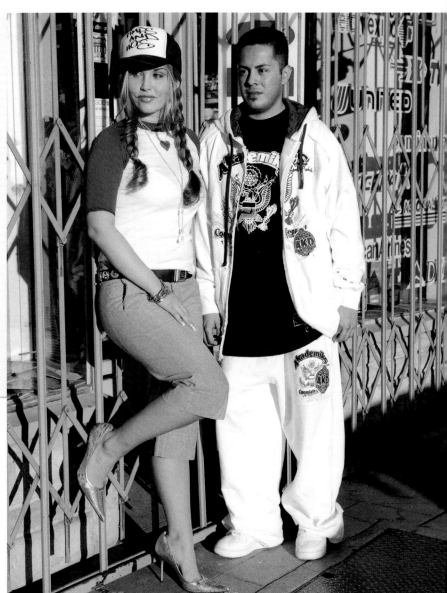

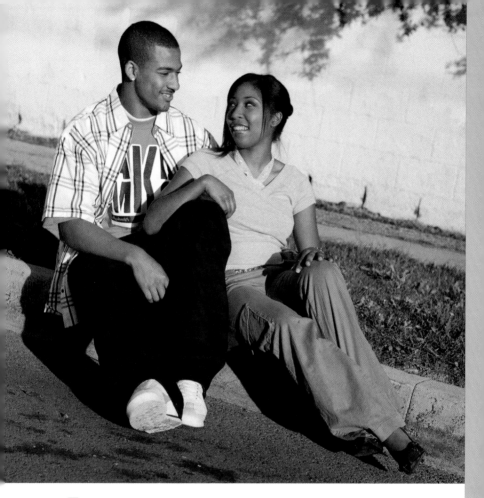

Layering is a great way to add another dimension to an outfit. Personally, I really like to put halter tops under lower-cut shirts.

PITCHER (left)

TRUCKER HAT: Beverly Hills
Pimps & Ho's
LONG NECKLACE: Gorjana
HEART NECKLACE: Lee Riot
TOP: Rojas
BRACELET: Kenneth Cole
BELT: Little Earth
PANTS: Hot Kiss
HEELS: Steve Madden

MISS FIT (right)

HALTER: Forever 21
SWEATSHIRT: Forever 21
BRACELET: Amber's Escapades
CHARM BRACELET: Lee Riot
BELT: Leatherock
PANTS: Forever 21
HEELS: Ecko Red

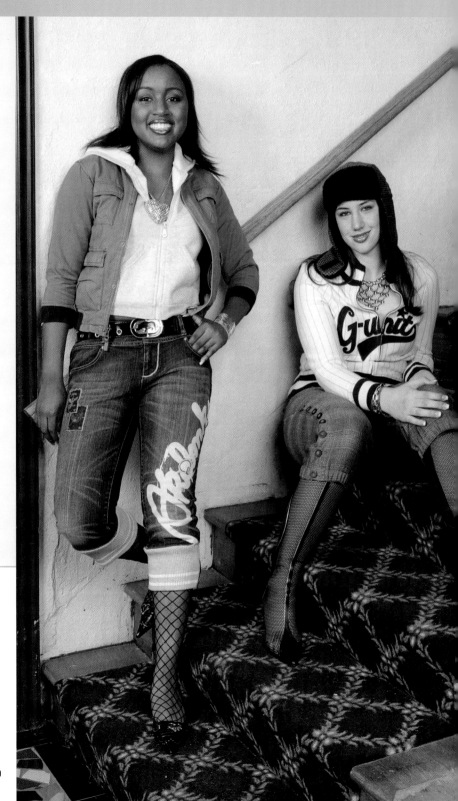

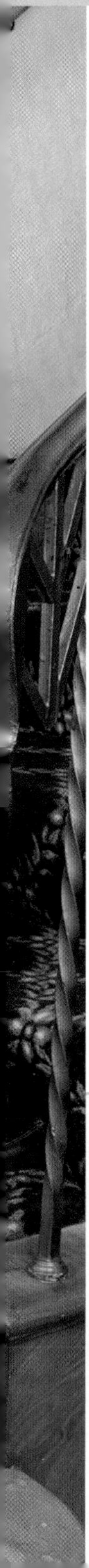

Capris, Bermuda shorts, and ripped pants all work well with fishnets. Gray is generally regarded as boring, but if you glam up a sweatshirt and other casual garments you can really expand your wardrobe.

TRAILER PARQUE (left)

NECKLACE: Sleaze
JACKET: Target
ZIP-UP HOODIE: Roxy
BELT: Ecko Red
PANTS: Akademiks
FISHNETS: dance shop
HEELS: Steve Madden

DEFURREL (right)

HAT: Bloomingdale's
NECKLACE: Marianna's Designer Jewelry
ZIP-UP JACKET: G Unit
BRACELET: Kenneth Cole
PANTS: G Unit
BOOTS: Michael Antonio

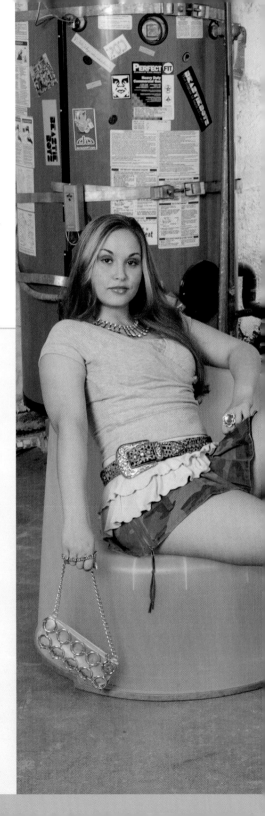

I really like the color combination of blues and olive green. Also, I've always felt like if you're wearing a big necklace, leave the earrings at home.

RETRO SPECT (left)

NECKLACE: Marianna's Designer Jewelry

TANK: Forever 21

SWEATSHIRT: Forever 21

RING: Marianna's Designer Jewelry

BELT: Leatherock

HANDBAG: Guess

SKIRT: Forever 21

TENNIS SHOES: Converse

HAFNIUM (right)

HAT: Forever 21

NECKLACE: Marianna's Designer Jewelry

JACKET: Forever 21

HALTER: Forever 21

CLUTCH: Forever 21

BELT: Leatherock

WORKOUT GLOVES: Bello

PANTS: Forever 21

BOOTS: Steve Madden

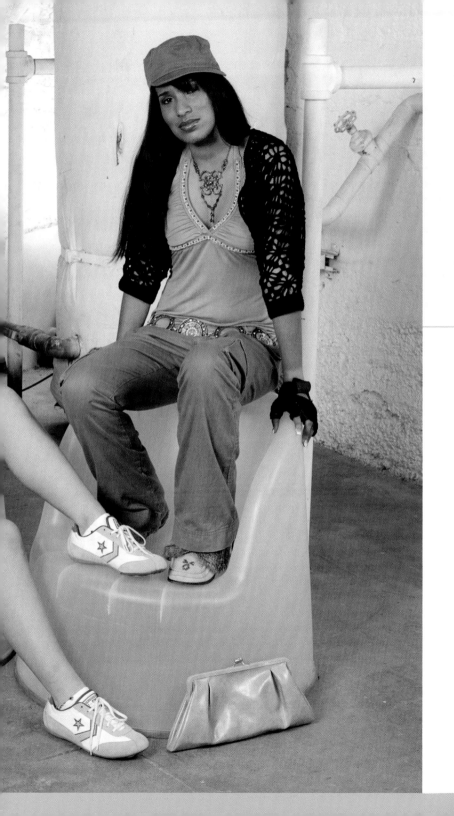

You'll be amazed at how taking some generally conservative pieces and fabrics—and putting a spin on them—will help expand your wardrobe.

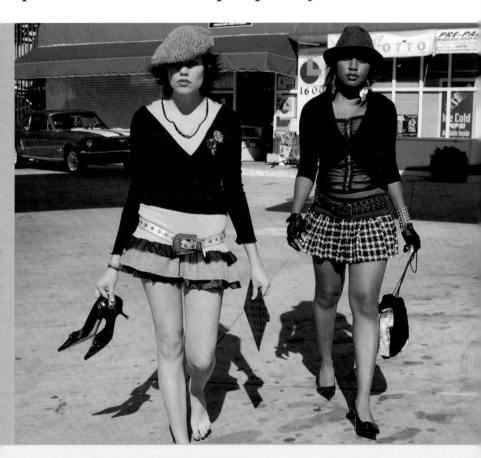

TWISTED CONSERVATIVE

TAINTED (left)

HAT: vintage

SWEATER: Forever 21

DRESS: Rojas

BROOCHES: Marianna's Designer Jewelry

CLUTCH: vintage Louis Vuitton

BELT: Leatherock

HEELS: Steve Madden

STUNT (right)

FEDORA: vintage

EARRINGS: Forever 21

TOP: Forever 21

BLAZER: Forever 21

BRACELET: Marianna's Designer Jewelry

WORKOUT GLOVES: Bello

PURSE: vintage

BELT: Wal-Mart

SKIRT: Rojas

HEELS: Ecko Red

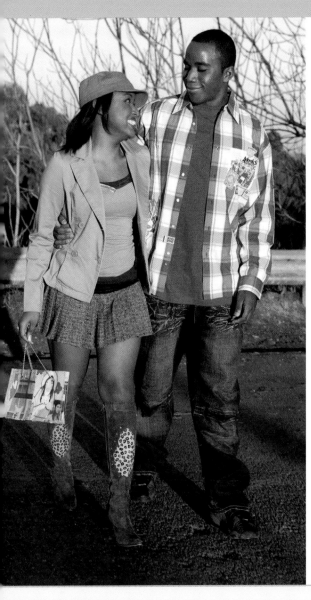

*B*lazers are definitely a must-have in every girl's wardrobe. They can go with a range of different bottoms and are a great piece with which to do some simple, but creative, layering.

FOND ELLE

MILITARY CAP: Peter Grimm Headwear
UNDERSHIRT: Forever 21
TOP: Forever 21
BLAZER: Forever 21
RING: Amber's Escapades
HANDBAG: Your Sister's Mustache
SKIRT: Rojas
BOOTS: Michael Antonio

Pointy toe shoes are always in style and investing in them is always a good idea. It's also a good idea to start looking at shoes on the more pricey side since they will last longer now that your foot has stopped growing.

WINDEX (left)

BEANIE: Bonknits by Bonnie
NECKLACE: Sleaze
BLOUSE: Hot Kiss
SHIRT: Forever 21
SEQUINED GLOVES: personal creation
BELT: Leatherock
PANTS: Forever 21
HEELS: Ecko Red

SRI LANKA (right)

MILITARY CAP: Peter Grimm Headwear
NECKLACE: Sleaze
HALTER TOP: Forever 21
BLAZER: Ecko Red
HANDBAG: Leatherock
BELT: Leatherock
PANTS: Forever 21
COWBOY BOOTS: Steve Madden

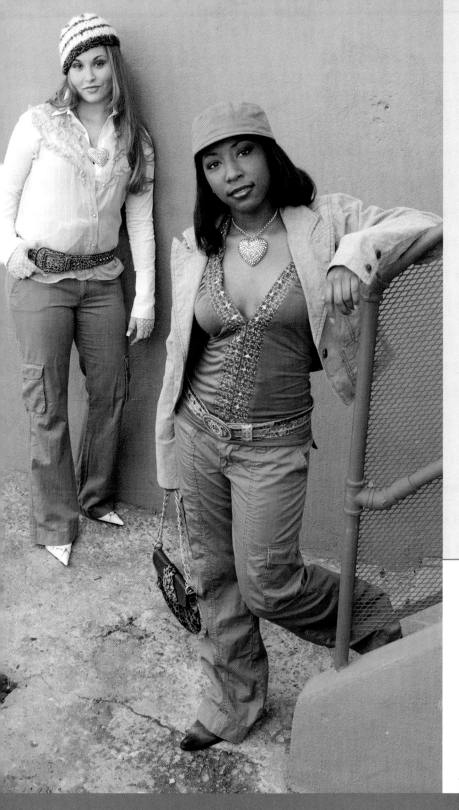

A white jacket or blazer is another must in every girl's wardrobe. Collars are very important and should always be adjusted before going out. It's up to you, but turning a collar up really adds spice to an outfit. As far as sleeve length goes, your two options are to leave your sleeves rolled down or roll them halfway up your forearm.

APHRODISIAC (left)

BRA: Marciano
TANK: Target
JACKET: Akademiks
BANGLES: inexpensive Indian boutique
BRACELET: Marciano
DENIM JEANS: Boom Boom Jeans
HEELS: Ecko Red

MYSTIC (right)

FEDORA: Peter Grimm Headwear
SHIRT: inexpensive boutique
BRACELET: Rampage
JACKET: Baba
SKIRT: Miken
BELT: garment district of Los Angeles
HEELS: Steve Madden

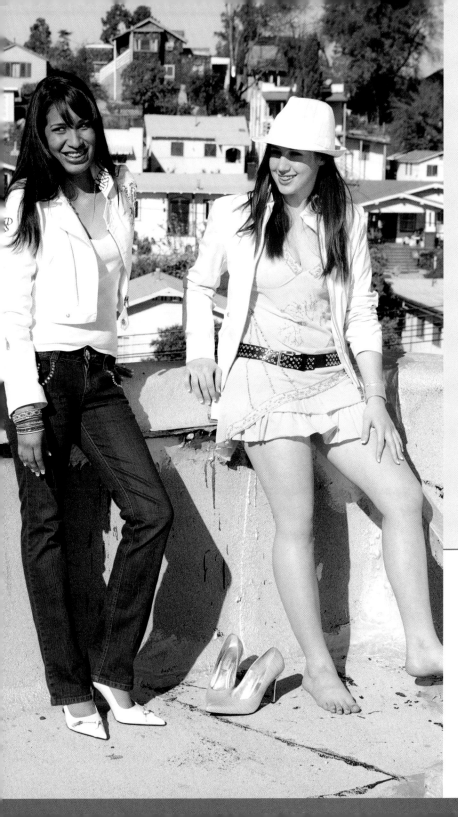

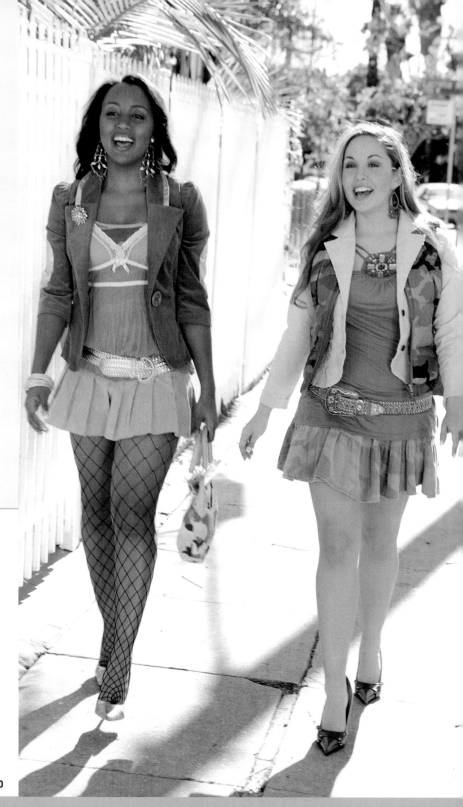

*W*hen wearing a short skirt, it's best to stay away from a low-cut shirt. All shirts—besides halter tops— pretty much look good with long earrings. Heels are important to have in your wardrobe. Also make sure that when you try them on you look at your whole leg instead of just your foot. Don't underestimate the fact that certain shoes and heels can be flattering or unflattering to your figure.

PEGAJOSO (left)

EARRINGS: Marianna's Designer Jewelry

BLAZER: Voom

BROOCH: Marianna's Designer Jewelry

TANK: Forever 21

TOP: inexpensive boutique

BRACELETS: Forever 21

HANDBAG: Forever 21

BELT: inexpensive boutique

SKIRT: Forever 21

FISHNETS: dance shop

HEELS: Steve Madden

SIMBA (right)

EARRINGS: Marianna's Designer Jewelry

VEST: Triple 5 Soul

BLAZER: Hot Kiss

TOP: Forever 21

BELT: Leatherock

RING: Amber's Escapades

SKIRT: Forever 21

HEELS: Ecko Red

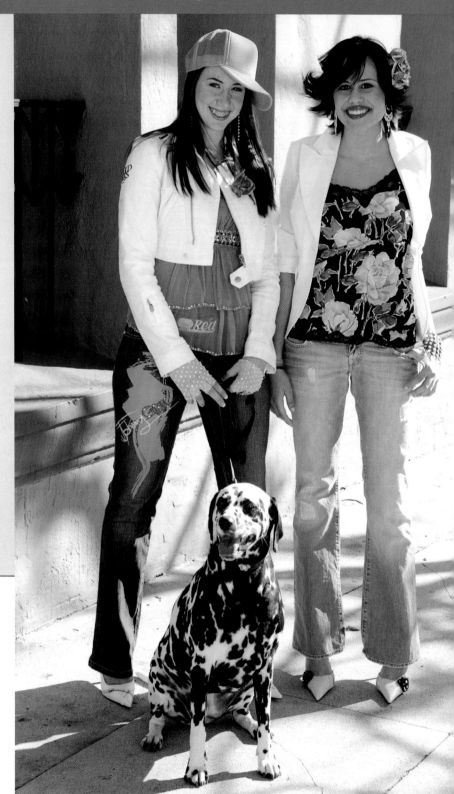

*S*houlder pads aren't always bad—
unless they're the ones from the '80s.
The jacket Nikki (right) is wearing has
a slight shoulder pad, which can give
your shoulders more shape. Shoulder
pads are great for all body types, unless
you are top-heavy.

DAY DREAM (left)

TRUCKER HAT: Beverly Hills Bookie
EARRINGS: Amber's Escapades
JACKET: Akademiks
TOP: inexpensive boutique
FLOWER: Sleaze
SEQUINED GLOVES: personal creation
BELT: Ecko Red
DENIM JEANS: Johnny Girl
HEELS: Ecko Red

POISON INFLUENCE (right)

FLOWER: Sleaze
EARRINGS: Macy's
BLAZER: Forever 21
TOP: vintage
BRACELET: Marianna's Designer
Jewelry
DENIM JEANS: Lucky Brand Jeans
HEELS: Steve Madden

This shot is definitely one of my favorites. Vertical lines, like the ones in the pants that Angie (left) is wearing, help to elongate the legs. If you are worried about a plunging neckline revealing too much, you can wear a camisole or halter top underneath.

ASBESTOS (left)

TRUCKER HAT: Beverly Hills Pimps & Ho's

HALTER TOP: Hot Kiss

TUBE TOP: inexpensive boutique

PURSE: Leatherock

BRACELET: Marianna's Designer Jewelry

BELT: Leatherock

PANTS: Forever 21

BOOTS: Vitiare

CHINCHILLA (right)

NECKLACE: Marianna's Designer Jewelry

BIKINI TOP: Akademiks

SWEATER: Forever 21

SKIRT: Forever 21

BRACELET: vintage

BELT: Ecko Red

WORKOUT GLOVES: Bello

FISHNETS: dance shop

TENNIS SHOES: Converse

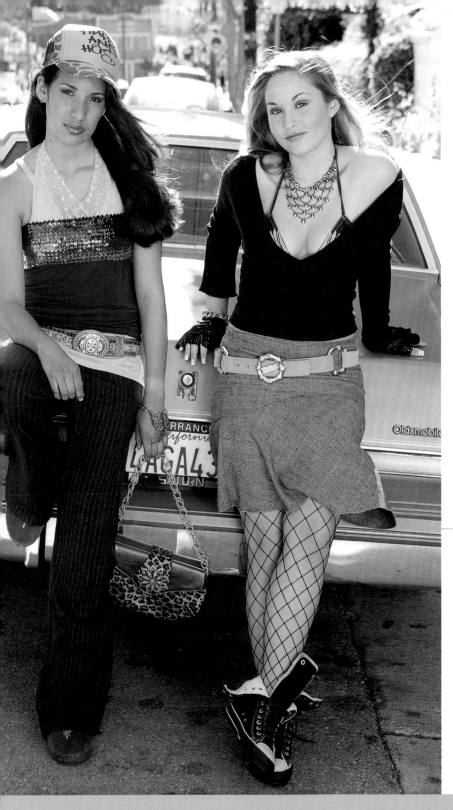

*W*hen wearing a short skirt, you can wear tights that hit mid-calf. This way your legs won't be as exposed.

MUSE (left)

EARRINGS: Rampage
SWEATER: inexpensive boutique
TOP: inexpensive boutique
BRACELET: Kenneth Cole
SKIRT: Hot Kiss
SPIDER: Marianna's Designer Jewelry
LEG WARMERS: Target
HEELS: vintage

TIGER LILY (right)

NECKLACE: Marianna's Designer Jewelry
BLAZER: Marciano
BROOCH: Marianna's Designer Jewelry
SWEATER: Rampage
TANK: inexpensive boutique
PURSE: Fetish
SKIRT: G Unit
BOOTS: Michael Antonio

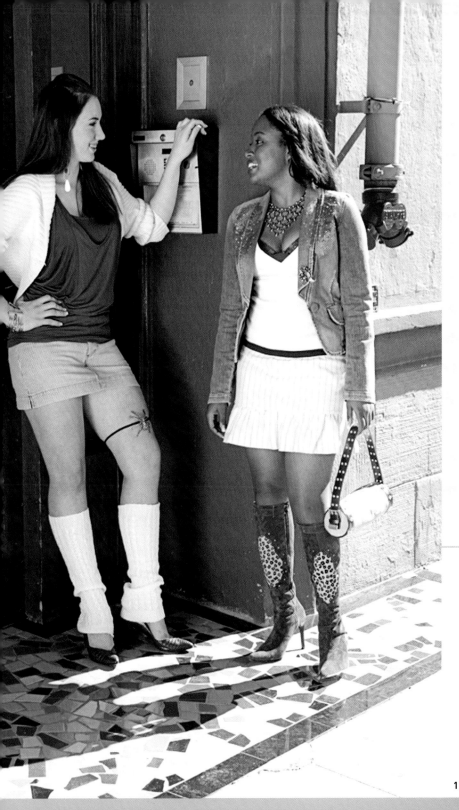

This is an example of an ensemble that plays off a single color. If you try this, always remember to include different shades and fabrics of the same color.

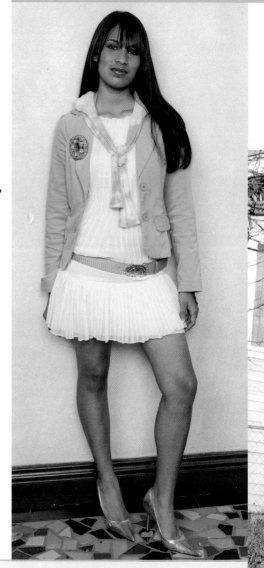

STRING BEAN (above)

TOP: Forever 21

BLAZER: Forever 21

DRESS: Rojas

BROOCH: vintage

BRACELET: Marianna's Designer Jewelry

BELT: Ecko Red

HEELS: Steve Madden

MARTIAN (right)

EARRINGS: Gorjana

NECKLACE: Gorjana

BRA: Chinese Laundry

TOP: Custo

BELT: Leatherock

PANTS: Forever 21

COWBOY BOOTS: Steve Madden

*P*ants with a flare at the bottom typically make your legs appear slimmer, because the width of the pants across your thigh is the same as the width across your ankle.

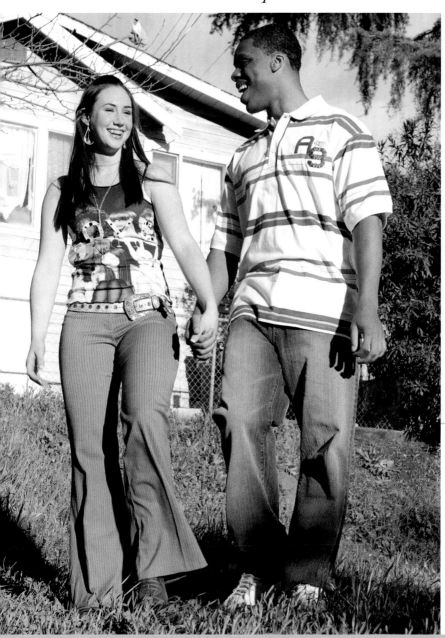

*R*emember that wearing brooches in clusters is good. Accessorizing with two or more (depending on the size) looks more interesting than one on its own. Wear thigh jewelry if you're looking for something a little different than the typical accessory. But avoid wearing thigh jewelry if you don't want people to look directly at your legs.

VANILLA (left)

BLAZER: Forever 21

BROOCHES: Marianna's Designer Jewelry

TOP: vintage

BRACELET: Rampage

HANDBAG: Marciano

BELT: Fetish

DENIM JEANS: Lucky Brand Jeans

HEELS: Michael Antonio

TINKER BELL (right)

EARRINGS: Marianna's Designer Jewelry

SHIRT: Triple 5 Soul

BRACELET: vintage

PINK BRACELET: Forever 21

SKIRT: Akademiks

SPIDER: Marianna's Designer Jewelry

LEG WARMERS: Target

HEELS: Steve Madden

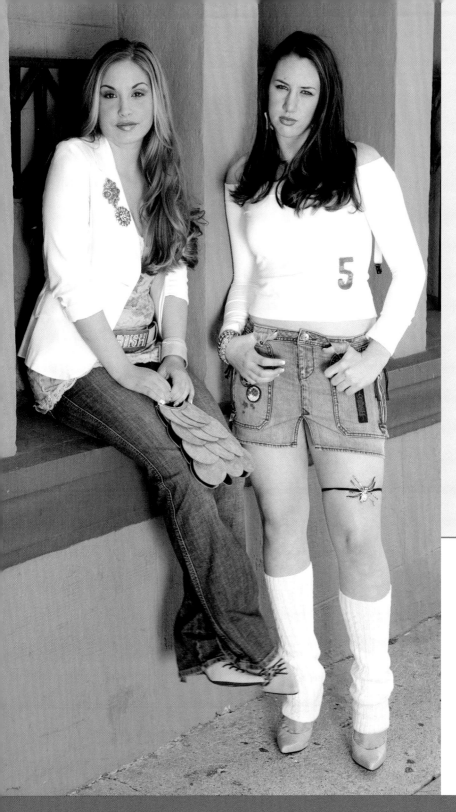

GLAM

LEMONADE (left)

FLOWER: Sleaze

SUNGLASSES: garment district of Los Angeles

EARRINGS: Amber's Escapades

NECKLACE: Marianna's Designer Jewelry

TRENCH COAT: Hot Kiss

DRESS: Hot Kiss

HANDBAG: Forever 21

HEELS: Steve Madden

5TH AVENUE (center)

FLOWER: Sleaze

SUNGLASSES: garment district of Los Angeles

TRENCH COAT: Hot Kiss

DRESS: Hot Kiss

HANDBAG: garment district of Los Angeles

SEQUINED GLOVES: personal creation

HEELS: Michael Antonio

CRAYOLA (right)

FLOWER: Sleaze

EARRINGS: Marianna's Designer Jewelry

SUNGLASSES: garment district of Los Angeles

TRENCH COAT: Hot Kiss

DRESS: Hot Kiss

BRACELETS: Forever 21

CLUTCH: Forever 21

FISHNETS: dance shop

SHOES: Michael Antonio

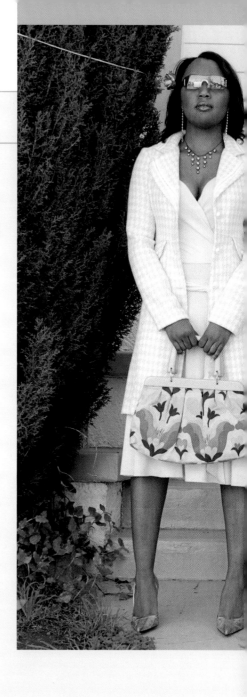

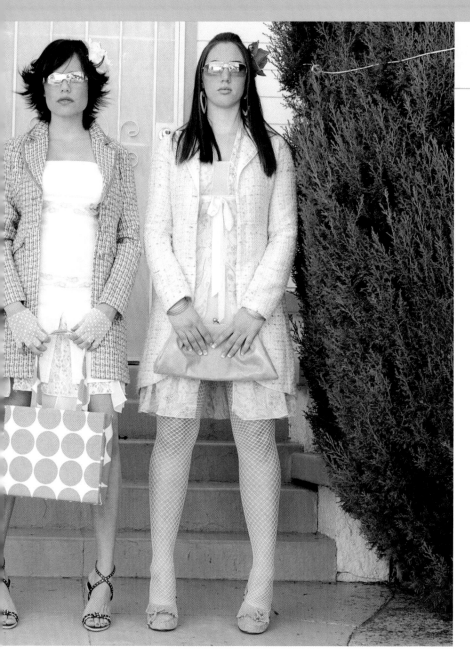

Mid-length trench coats are a great piece for the fall, and work on every body type. However, in any other season except fall and winter, trench coats tend to look ridiculous.

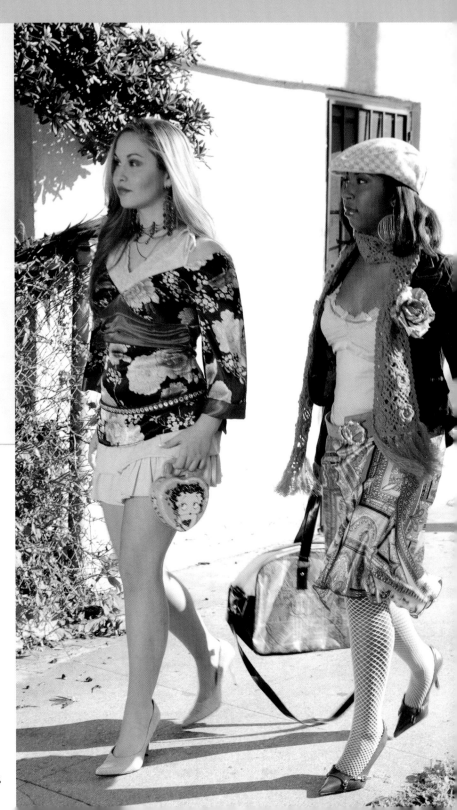

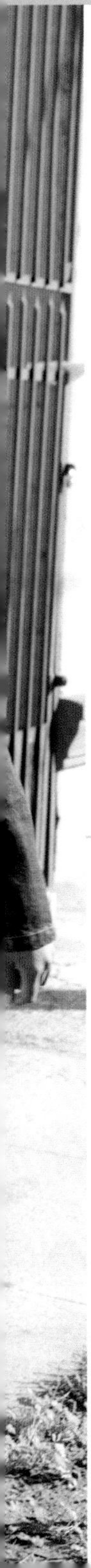

Here's an example of some great use of patterns (in the top on the left and the skirt on the right). When wearing patterns it's best that your other pieces are solid colors. This way you won't be all over the place.

ORIENT (left)

EARRINGS: Marianna's Designer Jewelry

NECKLACE: Marianna's Designer Jewelry

UNDERSHIRT: Hot Kiss

TOP: Forever 21

PURSE: personal creation

BELT: Leatherock

SKIRT: Miken

HEELS: Steve Madden

LILAC SUFFUSION (right)

DRIVER CAP: Forever 21

EARRINGS: Amber's Escapades

SCARF: Forever 21

FLOWER: Sleaze

BLAZER: Triple 5 Soul

TOP: Forever 21

BELT: Ecko Red

DUFFLE BAG: New York City Subway Line

SKIRT: Forever 21

FISHNETS: dance shop

HEELS: Ecko Red

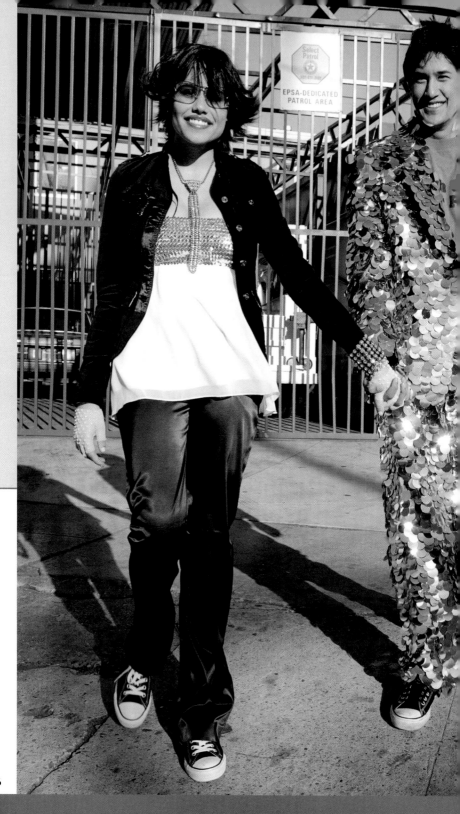

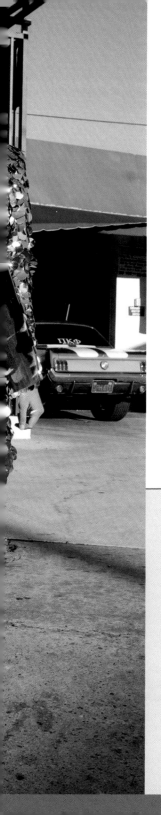

*B*lack and white Chuck Taylor Converse sneakers are an essential for every girl's wardrobe. Also, try to find unique or vintage jewelry like the necklace Nikki (left) is wearing to add some spiciness.

HADES

SUNGLASSES: garment district of Los Angeles

NECKLACE: vintage

JACKET: Triple 5 Soul

TOP: Forever 21

BRACELET: Marianna's Designer Jewelry

SEQUINED GLOVES: personal creation

PANTS: Hot Kiss

TENNIS SHOES: Converse

These two outfits are a bit on the simple side compared to other outfits in this book. However, when you decide to go with a simpler ensemble, make sure the top has a unique cut and quality fabrication.

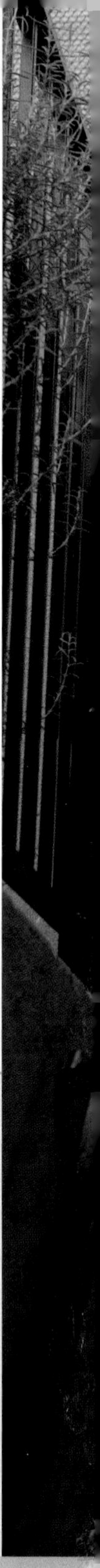

EGYPTIAN VIOLET (left)

NECKLACE: Marianna's Designer Jewelry

TOP: inexpensive boutique

DENIM JEANS: Lucky Brand Jeans

BRACELET: Marciano

RING: Marianna's Designer Jewelry

SPIDER: Marianna's Designer Jewelry

HEELS: Michael Antonio

BUTTERFLY (right)

EARRINGS: Marianna's Designer Jewelry

TOP: Marciano

BRACELET: Marianna's Designer Jewelry

PANTS: Johnny Girl

SHOES: Michael Antonio

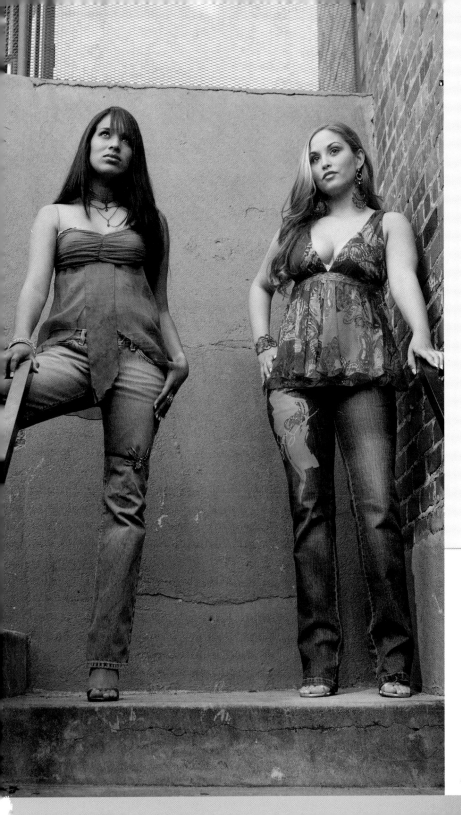

If you don't own Bermuda shorts, you can achieve that same look by cuffing pants at or above the knee. Bandanas are also a great accessory to play around with. Just remember, when tying a bandana make sure to tie it over your hair, not underneath.

MILITAIRE ELEGANTE
(left)

MILITARY CAP: Peter Grimm Headwear
EARRINGS: Amber's Escapades
TOP: Hot Kiss
JACKET: Triple 5 Soul
BRACELET: Marciano
BELT: Ecko Red
PANTS: Hot Kiss
HEELS: Michael Antonio

PINK PIRATE (right)

BANDANNA: EOEO
NECKLACE: Lee Riot
TOP: Custo
BRACELET: Lee Riot
BELT: Ecko Red
SHORT PANTS: Hot Kiss
SHOES: Michael Antonio

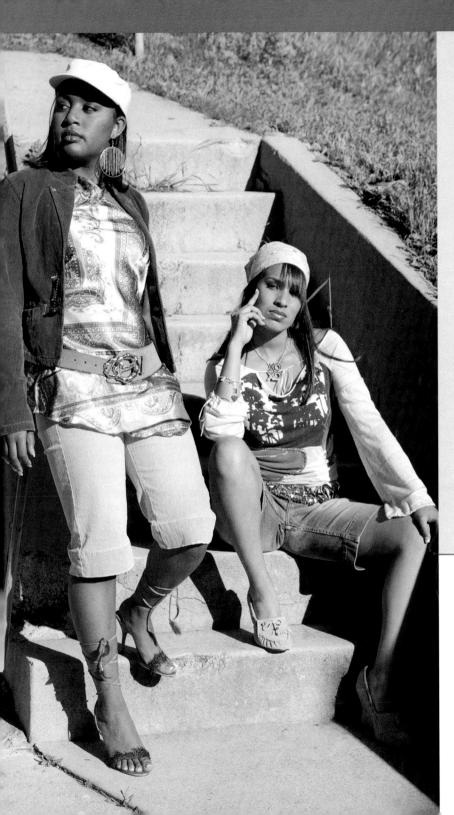

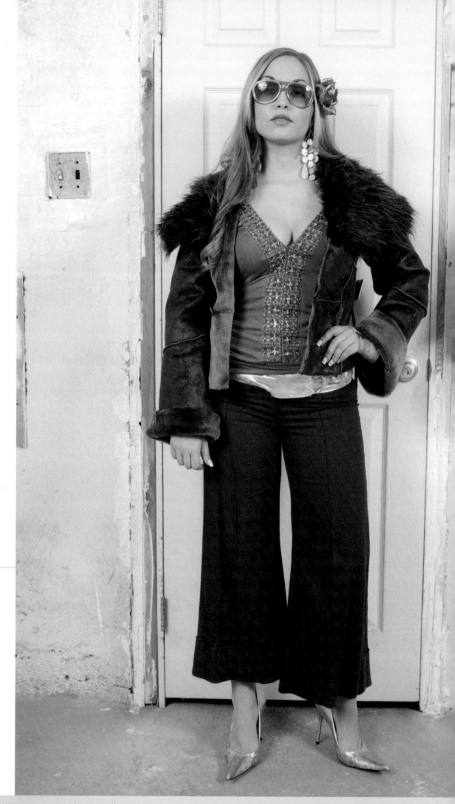

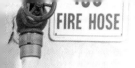

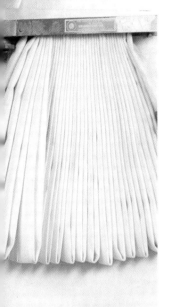

This is another example of the single-color look. If you are uncomfortable with your stomach and hip area, I suggest that you do not wear thick belts like the one Jackie is wearing. When dealing with gold accessories, make sure to use them in moderation and not to go over the top, or else it looks tacky.

PRIMA DONNA

SUNGLASSES: Rite Aid
FLOWER: Sleaze
EARRINGS: Rampage
JACKET: Paparazzi
TOP: Forever 21
BRACELET: Macy's
PANTS: Voom
SHOES: Steve Madden

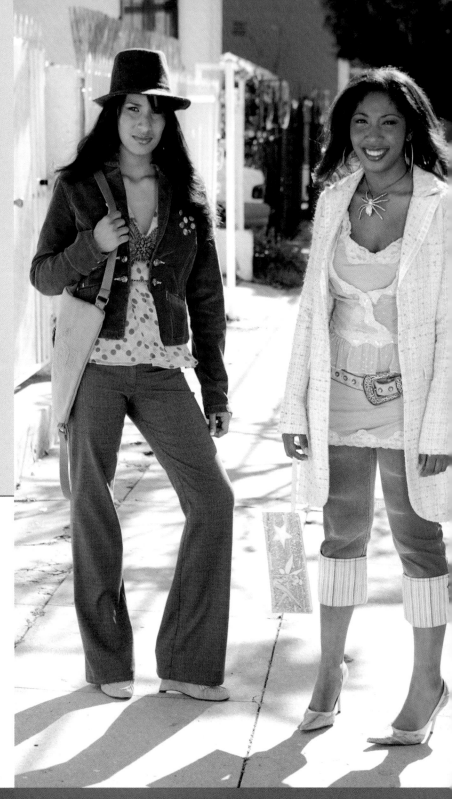

Long tops like the one Angie (left) is wearing, and even longer tops like the one Aviona (right) is wearing, are great for layering. Also, remember, when wearing a shorter jacket, balance it out by wearing a longer top.

ERA (left)

FEDORA: Forever 21
TOP: Voom
JACKET: Triple 5 Soul
PURSE: Ecko Red
PANTS: Forever 21
SHOES: Michael Antonio

DAWN (right)

EARRINGS: Forever 21
NECKLACE: Marianna's Designer Jewelry
TRENCH COAT: Hot Kiss
TANK: Forever 21
TOP: Forever 21
HANDBAG: Your Sister's Mustache
BELT: Leatherock
PANTS: Akademiks
HEELS: Steve Madden

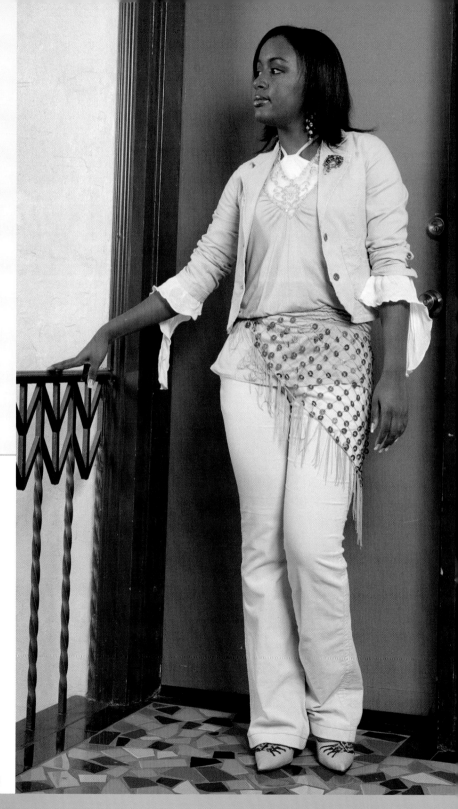

Khaki is a classic color choice that can be worn with an array of colors, and, of course, itself. Also, this is a good place to remind you that your shoes should always be darker than the rest of your outfit.

HERA

EARRINGS: Marianna's Designer Jewelry

UNDERSHIRT: vintage

TOP: Hot Kiss

BLOUSE: Charlotte Russe

BLAZER: Hot Kiss

BROOCH: Marianna's Designer Jewelry

SARONG: inexpensive boutique

PANTS: Forever 21

HEELS: Michael Antonio

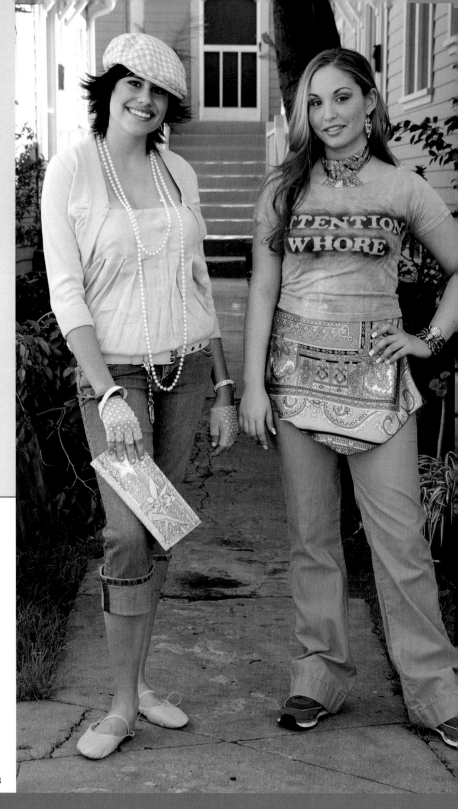

*W*ith these two outfits, as well as others, I wound up making one a little more feminine and the other a little more masculine. Try to figure out which is which. A good way to put a twist on a normal T-shirt is to cut it into an off-the-shoulder shirt and wear a halter underneath like Jackie (right) is wearing. Also, ballet flats are a trendy and comfortable way to get away from wearing your average tennis shoes.

SALLY (left)

DRIVER CAP: Forever 21
PEARLS: Rite Aid
TOP: vintage
SWEATER: Forever 21
BRACELETS: Amber's Escapades
HANDBAG: Your Sister's Mustache
BELT: Ecko Red
PANTS: Forever 21
SLIPPERS: dance shop

ATTENTION GRABBER (right)

EARRINGS: Lee Riot
TOP: Hot Kiss
T-SHIRT: Patrick Santa Ana
BRACELET: Marianna's Designer Jewelry
PANTS: Forever 21
TENNIS SHOES: Ecko Red

Perfect for school or going out with friends, this outfit is fashionable, comfy, and a tad sexy.

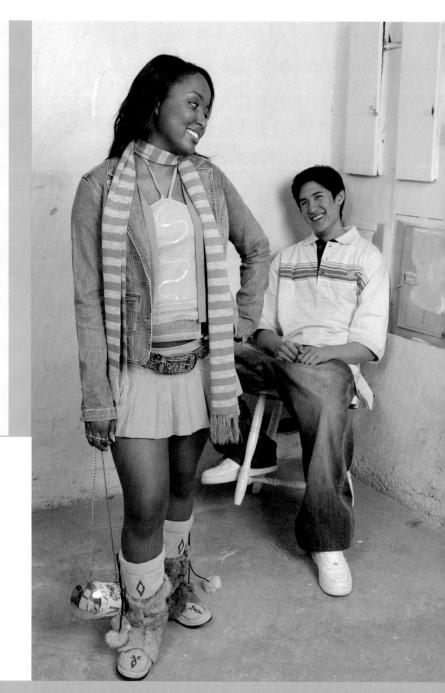

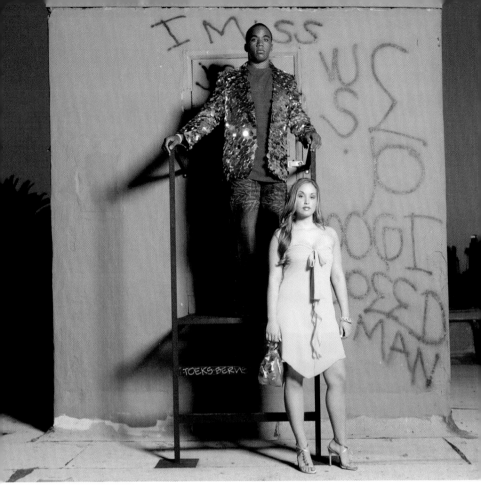

Going formal is simple—a dress, heels, and some fabulous accessories and you're ready to go!

ALUMINUM (left)

SCARF: Forever 21
TOP: vintage
CARDIGAN: Forever 21
BLAZER: Hot Kiss
PURSE: Little Earth
BELT: Leatherock
SKIRT: Forever 21
BOOTS: Steve Madden

SATURN (above)

EARRINGS: Marianna's Designer Jewelry
DRESS: Hot Kiss
BRACELET: Marciano
HANDBAG: inexpensive boutique
HEELS: Michael Antonio

When wearing things that are country-inspired, do not wear too many pieces from the same genre, like a cowboy hat, a cowboy belt buckle, a button-up country shirt, and cowboy boots. That's simply overkill. Also, long skirts are a great alternative to pants—not every skirt has to be a mini.

OKLAHOMA (left)

COWBOY HAT: Peter Grimm Headwear
EARRINGS: Macy's
SCARF: Forever 21
POLO SHIRT: Forever 21
TOP: Forever 21
BRACELET: Amber's Escapades
BELT: Leatherock
SKIRT: vintage

IRIS (right)

SCARF: Forever 21
BROOCHES: Marianna's Designer Jewelry
BLAZER: Voom
TOP: Hot Kiss
BELT: Leatherock
SKIRT: Forever 21
COWBOY BOOTS: Steve Madden

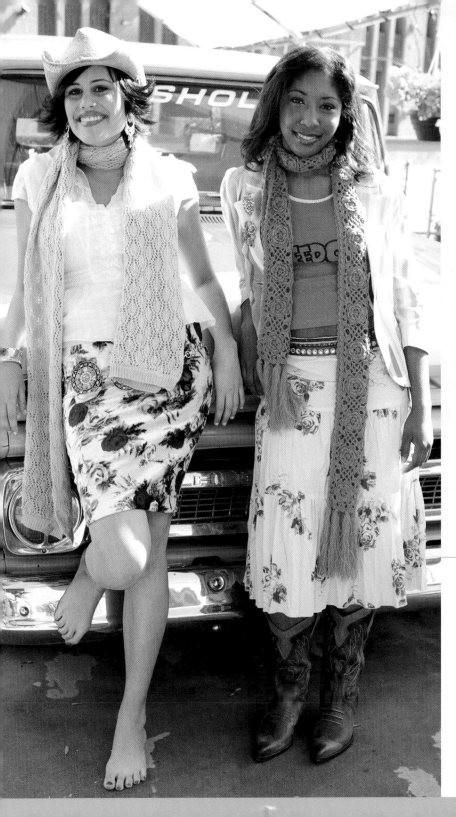

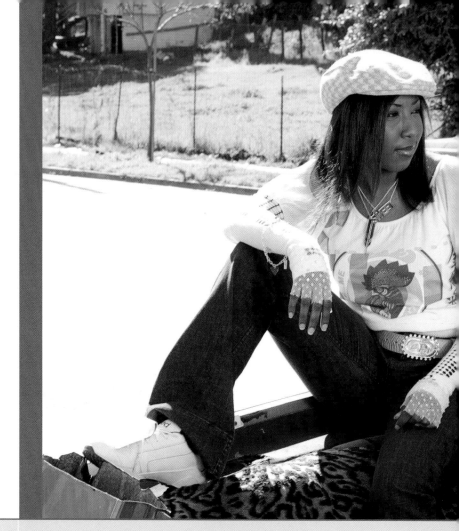

FUN

BLIZTER (left)

DRIVER CAP: Forever 21
NECKLACES: Lee Riot
TOP: Custo
BRACELET: Lee Riot
SEQUINED GLOVES: personal creation
BELT: Ecko Red
DENIM JEANS: Hot Kiss
TENNIS SHOES: Ecko Red

RAZZLE (right)

EARRINGS: Lee Riot
NECKLACES: Lee Riot
TOP: Custo
CHARM BRACELET: Lee Riot
BRACELET: Amber's Escapades
PANTS: Hot Kiss
TENNIS SHOES: Converse

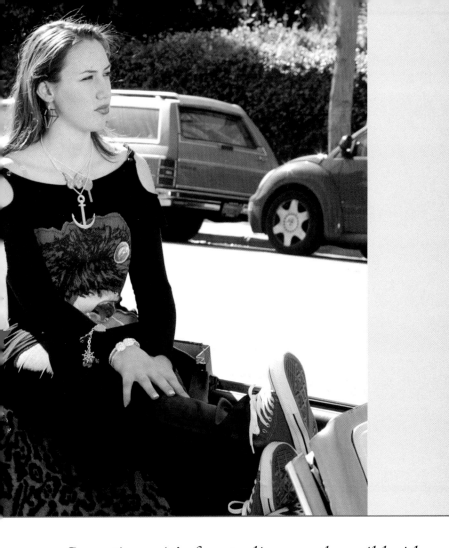

Sometimes it's fun to live on the wild side and dress in something completely crazy. Wearing multiple necklaces and bracelets always spices up an outfit. Keep in mind that it isn't such a good idea to wear a bandana or hat while driving around in a convertible, unless it's snug on your head or you're driving really slow.

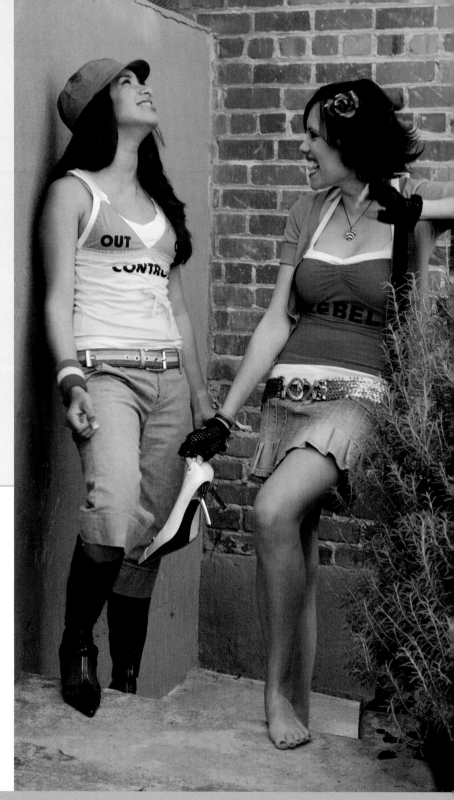

*M*ake sure to wear a strapless bra with any halter top or tube top, otherwise the showing straps look tacky and take away from the outfit. Although skirts aren't really worn until warm weather anyway, wearing a shrug, like the one Nikki (right) is sporting, will give you just a little added warmth if you need it and adds to the outfit as well.

CONTROL FREAK (left)

MILITARY CAP: Peter Grimm Headwear
WIFE-BEATER: Target
TANK: Hot Kiss
WRISTBAND: Claire's
BELT: Ecko Red
PANTS: Hot Kiss
BOOTS: Michael Antonio

REBELLIOUS JULY (right)

FLOWER: Sleaze
NECKLACE: Marianna's Designer Jewelry
SHRUG: Forever 21
HALTER TOP: Hot Kiss
WORKOUT GLOVES: Bello
BELT: Ecko Red
SKIRT: Akademiks
HEELS: Ecko Red

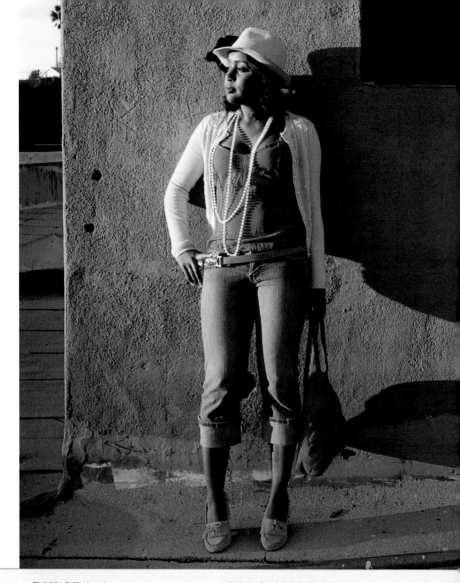

DULCE (left)

FEDORA: Armani Exchange
PEARLS: Rite Aid
CARDIGAN: Lucky Brand Jeans
TOP: Lucky Brand Jeans
BELT: Ecko Red
HANDBAG: Forever 21
BRACELET: Marciano
JEANS: Forever 21
SHOES: Michael Antonio

SOUR APPLE (right)

TRACK JACKET: Miken
BLAZER: Voom
HALTER TOP: Forever 21
SCARF: Forever 21
CLUTCH: Forever 21
JEANS: Forever 21
TENNIS SHOES: Ecko Red

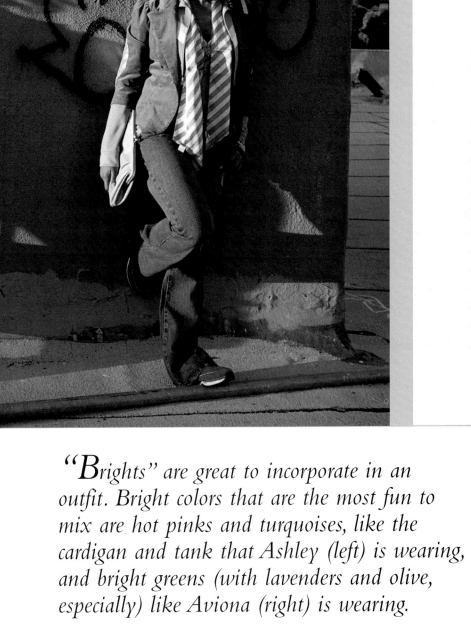

"Brights" are great to incorporate in an outfit. Bright colors that are the most fun to mix are hot pinks and turquoises, like the cardigan and tank that Ashley (left) is wearing, and bright greens (with lavenders and olive, especially) like Aviona (right) is wearing.

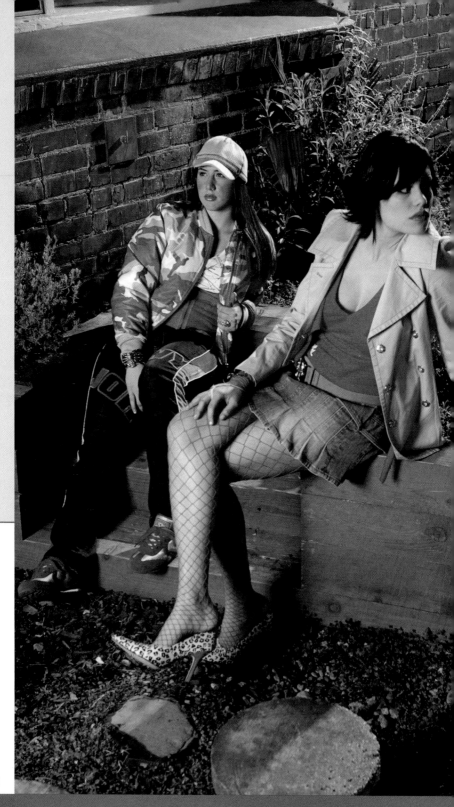

Make sure that when you wear a hat with a brim you're not wearing it too low over your eyes. You want to make sure that you can still see in front of you without having to tip your head up. When it comes to leopard print, colors in the brown family generally work best. But if you want to go bright, pinks are a great choice.

PINK KISS (left)

HAT: Peter Grimm Headwear
EARRINGS: Amber's Escapades
TANK: Amber's Escapades
ZIP-UP JACKET: Akademiks
BOMBER JACKET: Amber's Escapades
BRACELET: Marianna's Designer Jewelry
RING: Amber's Escapades
PANTS: Johnny Girl
TENNIS SHOES: Converse

STREET FLAMINGO (right)

TRENCH COAT: G Unit
TOP: Akademiks
ARMBAND: personal creation
BRACELET: Marianna's Designer Jewelry
BELT: Ecko Red
SKIRT: Akademiks
FISHNETS: dance shop
HEELS: Michael Antonio

If you are going to try to pull off lots of different patterns at the same time, make sure that the patterns are the same colors and not too similar.

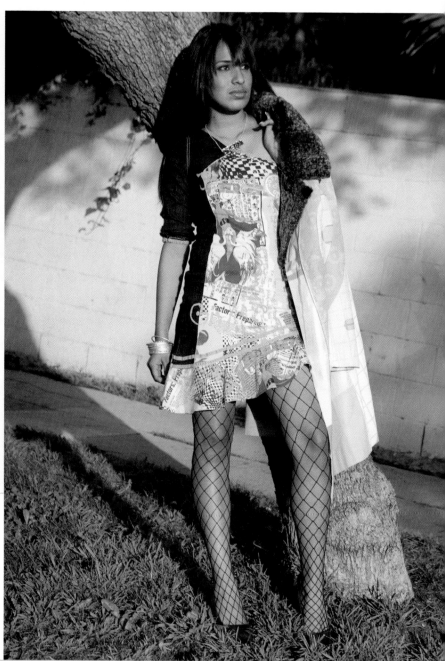

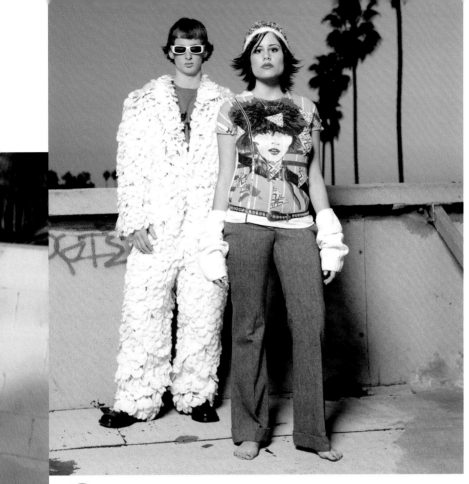

Continuing the same fabrication (or a similar fabrication) throughout an outfit often helps pull it all together. For example, Nikki (right) is wearing knit pants, her arm warmers are knit, and there are knit patches on her top.

ABSTRACT (left)

NECKLACE: Lee Riot
DRESS: Johnny Girl
COAT: Custo
BRACELETS: Forever 21
FISHNETS: dance shop
HEELS: Ecko Red

SOCK MONKEY (above)

BEANIE: Bonknits by Bonnie
NECKLACE: Lee Riot
TOP: Custo
ARM WARMERS: Target
BELT: Leatherock
PANTS: Forever 21

I love having fun with sweats. One way to keep your outfits with sweats from looking frumpy is by wearing a fitted top and glamming them up with accessories such as jewelry and scarves.

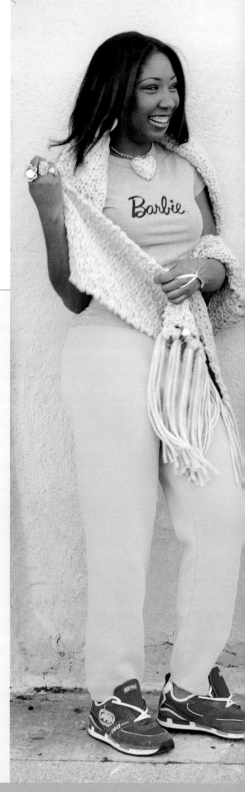

JUBILANT (left)

EARRINGS: Marianna's Designer Jewelry

SCARF: Lucky Brand Jeans

NECKLACE: Sleaze

T-SHIRT: Vintage Peanuts

GREEN RING: garment district of Los Angeles

PINK RING: Marianna's Designer Jewelry

BLUE RING: Marianna's Designer Jewelry

ARMBAND: personal creation

SWEATPANTS: Victoria's Secret

TENNIS SHOES: Ecko Red

TEASE (right)

EARRINGS: Marianna's Designer Jewelry

CHOKER: Marianna's Designer Jewelry

TOP: Victoria's Secret

BRACELET: Marianna's Designer Jewelry

SWEATPANTS: Victoria's Secret

TENNIS SHOES: Converse

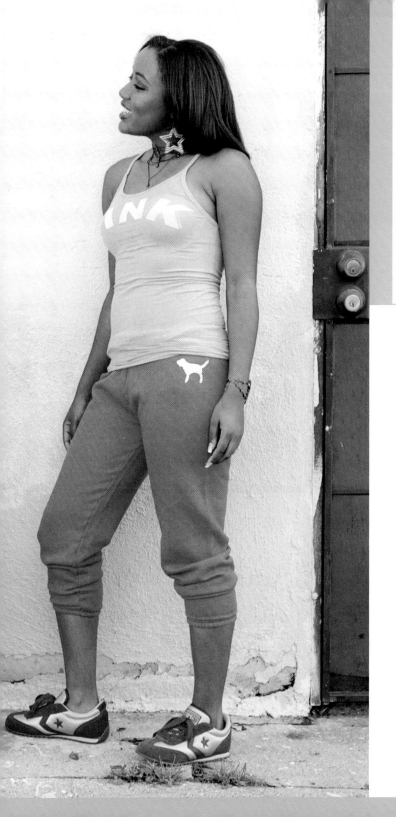

Hats, boots, or heels can completely change the look of an outfit. As compared, to say, the average tennis shoes, boots and heels usually make an outfit appear more dressy and fashionable.

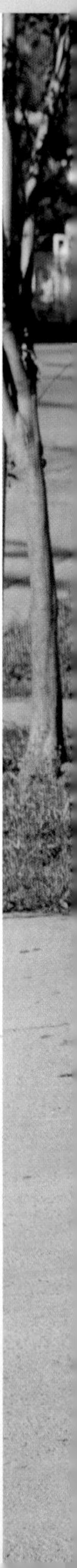

BUBBLE GUM TWIST (left)

TRUCKER HAT: Beverly Hills Pimps & Ho's

EARRINGS: Lee Riot

NECKLACE: Lee Riot

TOP: Custo

DRESS: Rojas

BRACELET: Lee Riot

BELT: Claire's

BOOTS: Steve Madden

FLEUR (right)

NECKLACE: Gorjana

BRA: Chinese Laundry

TOP: Custo

BROOCH: Marianna's Designer Jewelry

SKIRT: Rojas

HEELS: Steve Madden

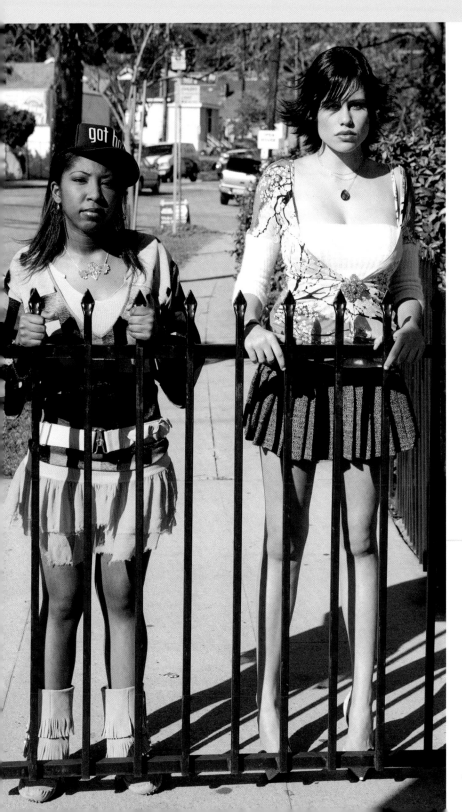

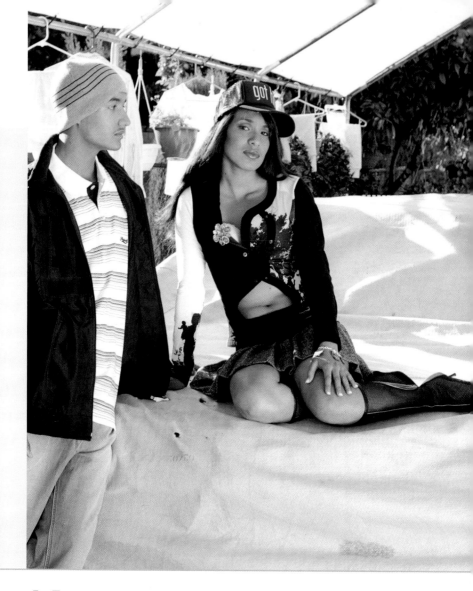

Not everyone can show off their belly, but if you are comfortable with your belly being exposed you can try shirts that have a unique cut, such as this one. Make sure that you do not expose too much cleavage though, otherwise you will give off a "skanky" impression.

This is more of an eclectic look that is military-inspired.

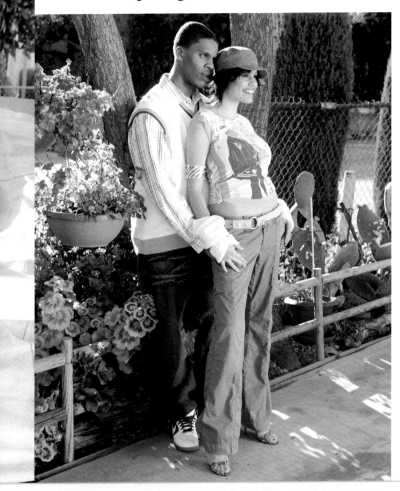

CINDERBLOCK (left)

TRUCKER HAT: Beverly Hills Pimps & Ho's

BRA: Chinese Laundry

TOP: Custo

BROOCH: Marianna's Designer Jewelry

BRACELET: Lee Riot

SKIRT: Rojas

BOOTS: Michael Antonio

NEMATODE (above)

MILITARY CAP: Peter Grimm Headwear

TOP: Custo

ARMBAND: Cheyne Hauk

ARM WARMERS: Target

BELT: Ecko Red

PANTS: Forever 21

HEELS: Michael Antonio

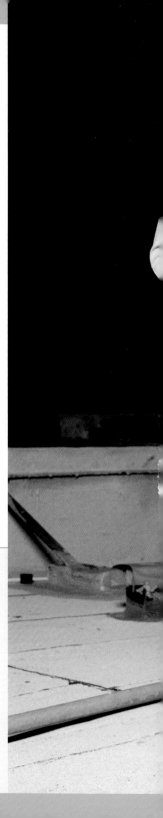

I love the way Carissa's (right) semi-elegant outfit contrasts with Spencer's casual style in this shot. A few quick ways to turn something from casual into something dressier is by wearing heels, tossing on a jacket or shrug, or adding a few accessories.

SECRETS

NECKLACE: Lee Riot
TOP: Chinese Laundry
COAT: Custo
BRACELET: Amber's Escapades
WORKOUT GLOVES: Bello
HEELS: Roach Killers

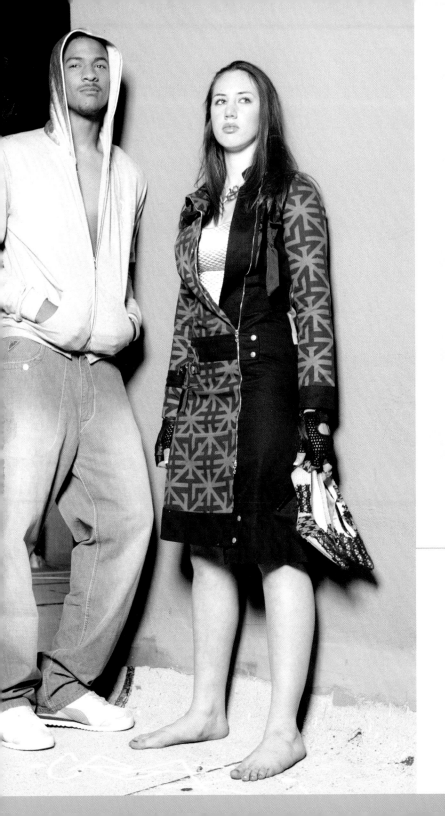

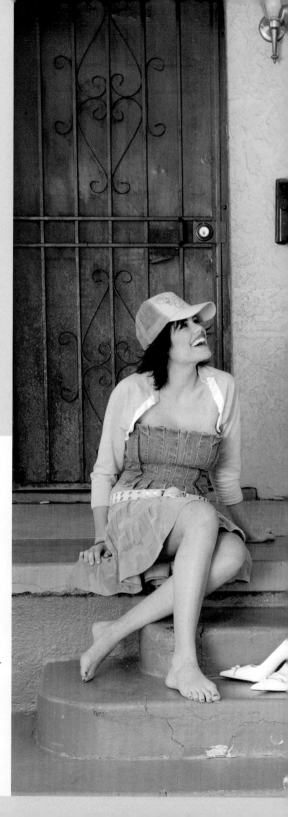

CALIENTE (left)

TRUCKER HAT: H&M
JACKET: personal creation
TOP: Akademiks
BELT: Ecko Red
SKIRT: Forever 21
HEELS: Ecko Red

PHARAOH (right)

BEANIE: Bonknits by Bonnie
BROOCH: Marianna's Designer Jewelry
NECKLACE: Marianna's Designer Jewelry
BIKINI TOP: Akademiks
DRESS: Juicy
BOOTS: Michael Antonio

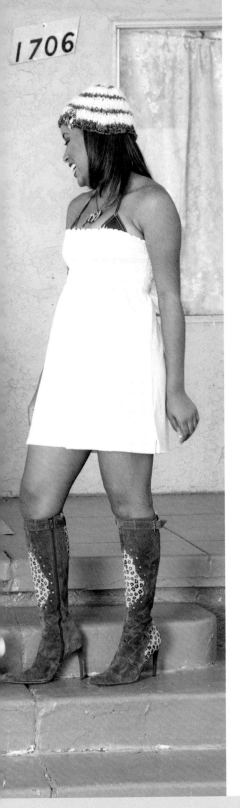

These outfits are intended for summer wear. The keys to putting a fashionable outfit together for warm weather is wearing light colors and exposing your legs. If you have tan lines that you don't want to be seen, avoid wearing tub tops. Or, consider wearing a shrug or cutting up a baseball top like the one Nikki (left) is wearing. Otherwise, if you can't hide your tan lines, it's just a way to show the world how tan you got in comparison to before!

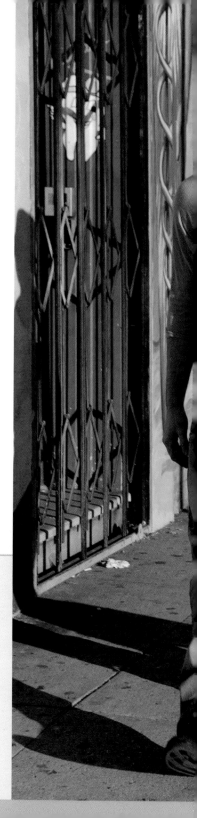

To keep flimsy tank top straps from slipping off your shoulders, try wearing a tank top with thicker straps underneath.

KARMA

COWBOY HAT: garment district of Los Angeles

UNDERSHIRT: Forever 21

TOP: Catch A Fire

BELT: Leatherock

DENIM JEANS: Forever 21

COWBOY BOOTS: Steve Madden

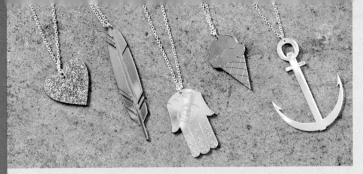

Lee Riot

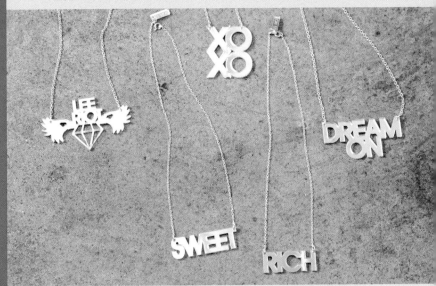

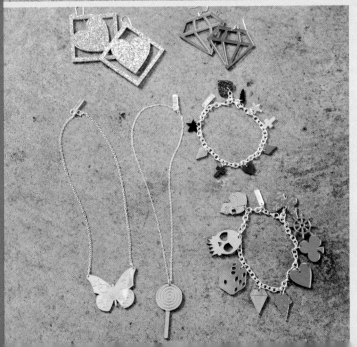

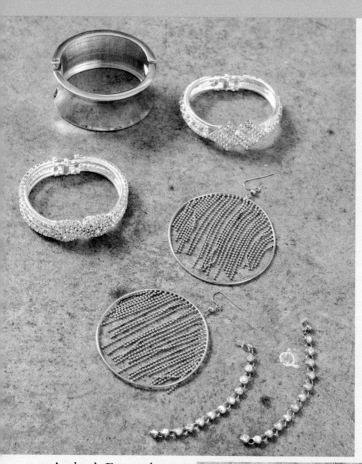

Amber's Escapades

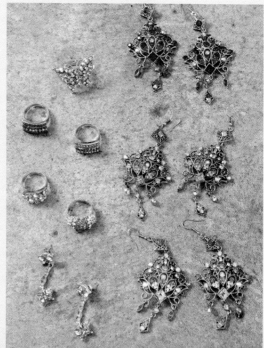

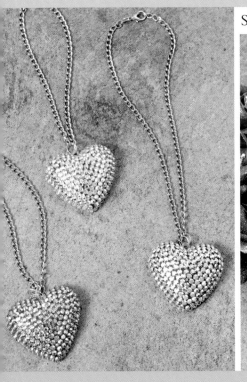

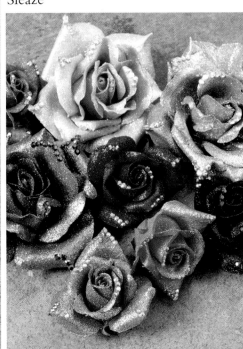

Sleaze

Cheyne Hauk

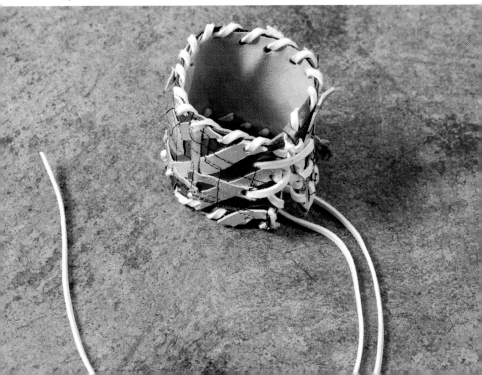

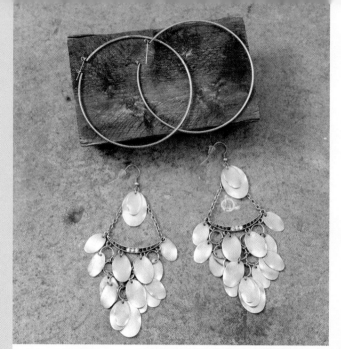

Forever 21

Chase's Personal
Collection

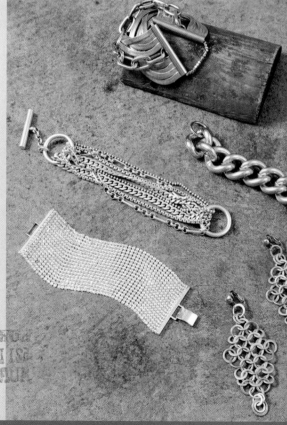

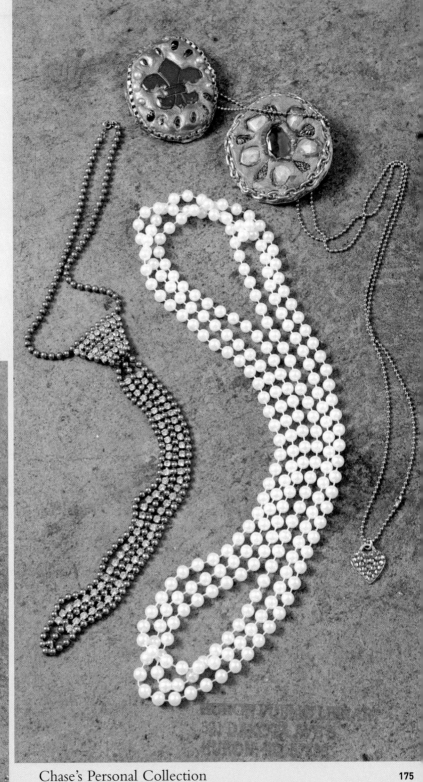

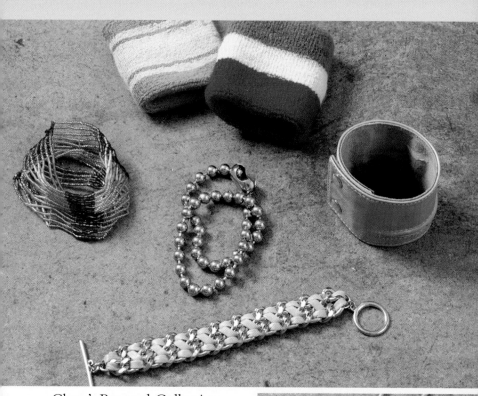

Chase's Personal Collection

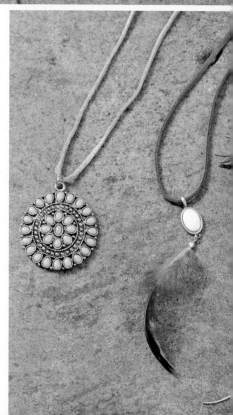

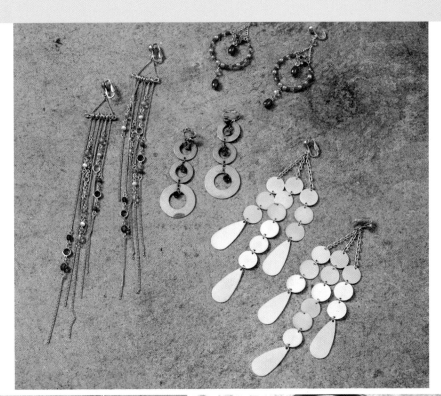

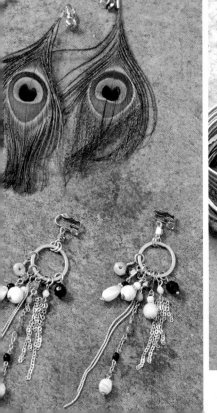

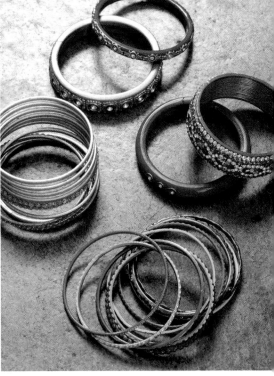

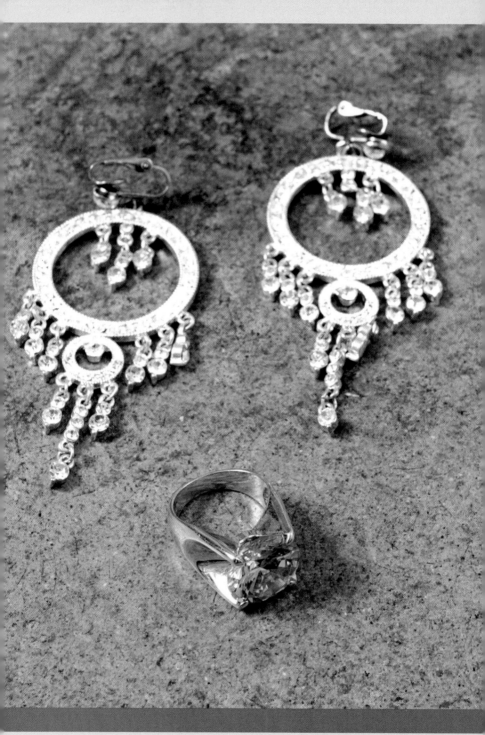

Chase's Personal Collection

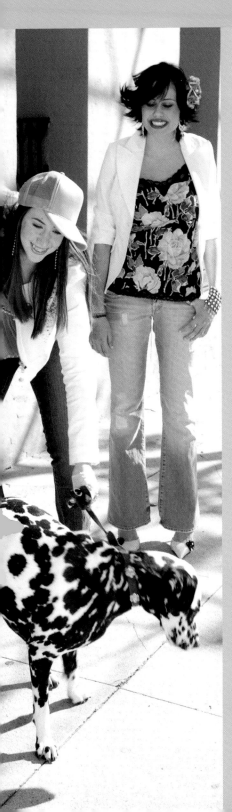

Part Three:
Where to Find It

9. Shop & Drop

Here's more about my favorite stuff—all the brands that are featured in this book—and where to get them. Check out the Web sites for more cool stuff and hot looks!

Top Manufacturers and Brands

Here are some of my favorites manufacturers and brands. You'll find quick ways to reach them in Yellow Pages on page 188.

★ **AKADEMIKS:** This company, established in 1999, makes very unique clothing that is carried in Macy's and Fred Segal, as well as smaller clothing chains. Akademiks is not only a hip-hop clothing line, but it also can be bought in different styles.

★ **AMBER'S ESCAPADES:** I love this brand for its great jewelry and shirts. All the shirts from Amber's Escapades are hand-painted and sport diva-chic slogans.

★ **AMERICAN RAG:** This line has some really cute pieces, like their blazers and skirts. American Rag is carried at Macy's in the junior's department.

★ **APPLE BOTTOMS:** Apple Bottoms is Nelly's clothing line for women. This line is carried in Macy's and makes extremely cute jeans. Apple Bottoms caters mostly to voluptuous girls.

★ **BABY PHAT:** This is a great hip-hop line, if that is your style. Baby Phat has a lot of really cute shirts, pants, skirts, and everything. These clothes fit girls who are voluptuous very nicely.

★ **BCBG:** See Top Stores on page 185.

★ **BELLA-CHIC TEASE:** This clothing line makes super-cute casual wear. What I love about them is that they have shirts that have a slogan in another language on the bottom of the shirt, and when you flip the shirt up, there is the translation.

★ **BEVERLY HILLS PIMPS & HO'S:** Worn by Gwen Stefani, Eminem, Ashton Kutcher, and Lenny Kravitz, this clothing line makes great hats, T-shirts, and sweats as well as customized leather jackets and hats.

★ **BIJOU DRIVE:** This jewelry company caters mostly to younger teens. Also, Destiny's Child has joined in support.

★ **BLUE MARLIN:** This clothing line is great. Blue Marlin makes a lot of cute casual tops that represent different sports teams. It's a predominantly hip-hop line, but it includes preppy genres as well. Blue Marlin is carried at Macy's and is pretty reasonably priced.

★ **BONGO:** This is a great inexpensive line that is carried at stores such as Charlotte Russe. One of my favorite things is their jeans.

★ **BONKNITS BY BONNIE:** These hand-knit pieces are adorable—beanies, scarves, fingerless gloves, shawls, all made from high-quality yarns in gorgeous color combinations.

★ **BOOM BOOM JEANS:** This jean company does great things with denim. Their pants make your butt look big in the hip-hop music-video girl way.

★ **CANDIES:** This company makes hot shoes for the younger teen.

★ **CATCH A FIRE:** This clothing line is designed by Bob Marley's daughter. I love Catch A Fire for its fun and unique clothing!

★ **CHEYNE HAUK:** A young up-and-coming jewelry designer, Cheyne Hauk has created some of the most unique pieces. I especially like his leather chokers and bracelets.

★ **CHICA:** This clothing line is another of my favorites. It's Latin inspired and makes really great tanks and T-shirts. Available at Sears, JCPenney, and www.drjays.com.

★ **CHICK BY NICKY HILTON:** Chick is a great juniors line that is affordable for all girls. The prices range from $25 to $125.

★ **CHINESE LAUNDRY:** This company makes fabulous shoes and lingerie as well as socks and stockings.

★ **CONVERSE:** Converse makes great tennis shoes; I especially like their classic Chuck Taylor All-Star low-tops in black.

★ **CUSTO BARCELONA:** Two genius designers created this label, located in Barcelona. Their clothing truly makes you feel like you are on the runway.

★ **DEMOSS JEANS:** This brand makes hot jeans that are reasonably priced. I especially like their tanks, which have décor on them.

★ **DOLLHOUSE:** This brand makes some great denim pieces as well as jackets. Dollhouse is sold at Wet Seal and Macy's.

★ **DORFMAN PACIFIC:** Dorfman Pacific is a hat line that produces many stylish hats.

★ **ECKO RED:** This brand is one of my favorites. I love everything from their shoes to their clothing to their accessories. Ecko Red is a hip-hop line, and what's great about them is that each season usually incorporates the same colors, and everything goes with everything else in the line, making styling fast and easy.

★ **ELAN:** This company makes clothing that reminds me of Juicy, but for a fraction of the price.

★ **EOEO:** This company is responsible for the Dear John letter T-shirts. What's great is that each T-shirt has its own authentic "Dear John" letter with it. The creator of this company, John Brown, saved his own Dear John letters from his past girlfriends, and he includes one on every tag.

★ **FETISH:** This clothing line is by Eve. What I really like about Fetish is that you could see Eve wearing the clothes in her line, unlike some other celebrity-owned lines. I particularly love the belts and purses.

★ **G UNIT:** This is a hot hip-hop clothing line. I really like the style of their jackets and coats.

★ **GANG RIO:** This company does a lot with denim and crystals. All the jeans are very pretty.

★ **GIRL STAR:** Girl Star has really cute purses as well as necklaces. This company also makes great bathing suits and skirts.

★ **GORJANA:** This new, up-and-coming jewelry designer has already been featured in numerous fashion magazines. I love her jewelry because it is absolutely gorgeous and just so delicate and feminine.

★ **GUESS:** See Top Stores on page 185.

★ **HOT KISS:** I love Hot Kiss! This label is a definite must-have in every girl's wardrobe. All the pieces are so feminine and high quality. I especially love the blazers—not to mention the reasonable prices.

★ **JAMES PERSE:** This clothing line is carried at Bloomingdale's. It is on the pricey side, but their shirts are made from extremely soft cotton—worth every penny! James Perse is a little more on the conservative side, but they do have some fabulous casual shirts.

★ **JET:** Jet produces tons of cute, simple shirts. It's usually carried at boutiques and is a little more on the expensive side.

★ **JOHNNY GIRL:** Johnny Girl is a hip-hop line and is a favorite of mine as well as the star of the Disney Channel's *That's So Raven*, Raven Symone. One thing that I really like about Johnny Girl is that a necklace comes with each garment. The line is reasonably priced and has matching shirts, jackets, pants, skirts, etc.

★ **JUICY COUTURE:** Everyone pretty much knows Juicy for their velour and terry cloth running suits. I love Juicy not only for their running suits but also for their new line of purses, as well as for their other clothing.

★ **JUNK FOOD FOREVER:** Junk Food makes hot casual attire, like purses and T-shirts. It's available at Kitson in Los Angeles.

★ **LEATHEROCK:** This company makes the most beautiful, extravagant belts, with studs, crystals, and fur. The purses are equally beautiful.

★ **LEE RIOT:** I love this jewelry line because the jewelry is like nothing I've seen before. Lee Riot makes earrings, necklaces, and bracelets out of Plexiglas as well as leather. Everything is so unique and fun! Lee Riot is carried at some boutiques in Los Angeles, like Rojas and Kitson. They also are starting a clothing line that makes fabulous blazers and tanks.

★ **LITTLE EARTH:** This company makes extremely unique purses and belts. I especially like their license-plate purses with Swarovski crystals and bottle-cap belts.

★ **LUCKY BRAND JEANS:** See Top Stores on page 185.

★ **MARIANNA'S DESIGNER JEWELRY:** See Top Stores on page 185.

★ **MECCA FEMME:** This line of clothing can be summed up with one word: breathtaking! Mecca Femme is feminine and sexy at the same time. Everything is high quality and simply beautiful. Mecca Femme is a little pricey, but if you're going to splurge, I would definitely encourage you to buy their clothing.

★ **MICHAEL ANTONIO:** These shoes are gorgeous! I love Michael Antonio shoes for their versatility, as well as how pretty they are. Every pair of shoes in the line is amazing. What's even better is that their shoes are even more than reasonably priced.

★ **MIGUEL TORRES:** Miguel Torres is incredible. He can create anything from clothing to accessories; he is the best!

★ **MIKEN:** Miken is traditionally known for their surf-chic wear. They just recently started making more fashionable items. I love their pieces for their versatility and comfort, as well as the reasonable pricing.

★ **MISS ME:** I love Miss Me jeans! They make great knock-offs of more upscale jeans like Juicy and Marciano. Of course, the quality isn't as good as the originals, but the price is great! A pair of jeans usually runs in the neighborhood of $50.

★ **N.A.I.:** I especially like N.A.I.'s Judith Leber–like purses—small handbags covered in crystals.

★ **NEW YORK CITY SUBWAY LINE:** I love this line for its great purses, duffel bags, T-shirts, and tanks. New York City Subway sports subway maps or subway numbers/letters on their pieces. It's hot casual wear that can be found at Virgin Megastores.

★ **OCEAN DRIVE CLOTHING:** I like this clothing line because it has the Juicy Couture flair, as well as some awesome tie-dyes.

★ **ORIENT EXPRESS:** The Orient Express line has gorgeous Asian-inspired clothing that is made from satin and has beads. It can be dressed up or dressed down. Wearing one of their pieces will definitely get you noticed.

★ **PETER GRIMM HEADWEAR:** The specialty hats that I like most from Peter Grimm Headwear are the hand-painted cowboy hats. They are amazing and so unique. Their other hats are also great!

★ **PICASSO STYLE INC.:** I really like this line because it is carried in so many places, from boutiques to clothing chains like Planet Funk. Picasso Style Inc., formally known as Picasso Style Jeans (PSJ), has some great pieces that are reasonably priced.

★ **PLANET BODY:** This company makes sexy casual wear. I really like this line because they make comfortable clothing that is also very stylish.

★ **PUSSYCAT:** Pussycat is a British line that I grew to like after seeing arrays of shirts that I thought were very cute.

★ **RAMPAGE:** This clothing line is carried in department stores such as Macy's. Rampage makes some great feminine pieces that are reasonably priced.

★ **ROACH KILLERS:** These custom-made shoes are one of a kind and super-hot!

★ **ROCAWEAR:** This is a great hip-hop juniors line. The line is a little more on the pricey side, but the quality is fantastic. Rocawear is a little tomboyish, but their clothing fits the curves nicely.

★ **ROJAS:** See Top Stores on page 185.

★ **SAN FRANCISCO CITY LIGHTS:** San Francisco City Lights manufactures some great pieces. The line is primarily casual chic, but everything is of the highest quality. You can purchase San Francisco City Lights at Bloomingdale's.

★ **SLEAZE:** Sleaze is an awesome line run by one woman. She makes the most beautiful crystal heart necklaces, as well as glitter, crystal rose pins, and hair pieces. I love Sleaze. Everything is absolutely beautiful!

★ **SPARKLICIOUS:** This is a line of shoes, jewelry, and watches that are completely covered in Swarovski crystals. Everything sparkles, just like the name.

★ **STEVE MADDEN:** See Top Stores on page 185.

★ **SUPER LUCKY CAT:** This clothing brand is amazing! Super Lucky Cat takes used clothing and creates fabulous new pieces. Super Lucky Cat retails in the neighborhood of $40 to $60. You can find Super Lucky Cat at Nordstrom's Brass Plum section or in Rampage.

★ **TEAM DIVA:** This company makes some of the most exquisite cowboy hats—from hats covered in crystals to patches.

★ **TIMBERLAND:** Timberland makes the greatest hiking boots. They come in all colors and are priced in a range from $90 to $150. Timberland was responsible for the trend with the high-heel hiking boots Beyonce Knowles wore in the '03 *Bonnie & Clyde* music video.

★ **TRIPLE 5 SOUL:** Triple 5 Soul is a great line and another one of my favorites. Their clothing is very versatile and can be mixed with hip-hop clothing as well as more feminine/preppy styles.

★ **VINTAGE PEANUTS:** I love their T-shirts! Vintage Peanuts T-shirts have been worn by celebrities like Hilary Duff and Jennifer Gardner and have been featured in many magazines. I especially like their Mickey T-shirts that come in so many different varieties. Also, the cotton is absolutely delicious.

★ **VITIARE:** This designer has the most awesome line of boots. They are a must-have in your wardrobe.

★ **WHITE BOY:** This company makes some great pieces. Some of their T-shirts are a little controversial, but definitely a must-have.

★ **XOXO:** This clothing brand is great. They make some fabulous shirts and jackets that are reasonably priced. XOXO is carried at Macy's junior's department.

★ **YOUR SISTER'S MUSTACHE:** Your Sister's Mustache has the most unique purses. I love them because the purses have pages out of magazines as the exterior as well as the interior. When I'm carrying one of those purses and I have downtime, I'll actually read the articles on the purse!

Top Stores

Here are some of my favorites stores. You'll find quick ways to reach them in Yellow Pages on page 188.

★ **ABERCROMBIE & FITCH:** I like A&F because they have cute, simple, comfy clothing. They make a lot of cute shirts that are great for layering, as well as some really great styles of jeans.

★ **AMERICAN EAGLE OUTFITTERS:** This clothing chain is a lot like Abercrombie & Fitch, but less expensive. American Eagle has a ton of cute T-shirts and always has a great summer line.

★ **BCBG:** This line is very feminine and is carried at Bloomingdale's as well as in their own chain of stores. BCBG has great pieces but is on the expensive side. If it's affordable for you, it's definitely a line to look for. If it isn't in your budget, don't sweat it.

★ **BEBE:** I really like Bebe because they sell great clothing for parties as well as casual occasions. Bebe is a little more on the pricey side, but you are sure to find high quality and unique clothing. Bebe's accessories, and of course their shoes and belts, are also fabulous!

★ **BIZ:** Located in Los Angeles, this company manages about four clothing lines. I especially like their outerwear and heavier jackets. Their clothing is also very reasonably priced.

★ **DIESEL:** This clothing line has amazing jeans as well as accessories. Diesel is expensive, but it's definitely worth it because it is so high quality.

★ **DOUGLAS FIR:** First and foremost, this is a guy's clothing line. So if you are looking for a gift to buy a boyfriend, this is a definite clothing store to hit, if you are located in the Los Angeles area.

★ **FOOT LOCKER:** Foot Locker carries tons of different shoes from Adidas to Converse to Timberlands. This chain also has tons of different baseball hats and jerseys.

★ **FOREVER 21:** This clothing chain carries a lot of trendy clothing and accessories that are extremely inexpensive. Go here for up-to-date trends without breaking your piggy bank. Forever 21's sister stores are XXI and Reference.

★ **GUESS:** Guess stands out in my mind for their quality and uniqueness, as well as for how feminine their styles are. I love this store (also their clothing line) because of all their great clothing, accessories, and shoes. Guess is a little more on the pricey side, but it's worth it! Guess can also be found in department stores.

★ **LUCKY BRAND JEANS:** I love Lucky Brand jeans! The fit is amazing, and there are so many different styles and washes. Lucky Brand is a little pricier, but definitely worth the splurge since their jeans are top quality. If there isn't a store near you, look for Lucky Brand Jeans in department stores.

★ **MACY'S:** The junior's department in Macy's carries everything from Rocawear, Akademiks, and Ecko Red to Roxy, XOXO, and Rampage. Their junior's jewelry, hat, and belt department is a one-stop shop.

★ **MARCIANO:** I can't even begin to explain how much I adore this line! Marciano is expensive, but walking into their store is priceless! Everything in the store is so beautiful that even if you do have a budget that can include a store like Marciano, it's hard to narrow the store's selection down to what you want to try on. Bottom line: Everything is amazing!

★ **MARIANNA'S DESIGNER JEWELRY:** Marianna works with Bob Mackie. Right there, that should let you know how amazing her stuff is. Marianna designs everything herself, and all the pieces in her boutique are gorgeous. All pieces are made with Austrian Swarovski crystals; celebrities like Cher have worn and own her jewelry. All her pieces are so sparkly and pretty. What I especially like is her trademark spider jewelry. Another thing that I like about Marianna's Designer Jewelry is that it is very affordable!

★ **NORDSTROM:** Nordstrom's junior's department, Brass Plum, has great clothing for teens. There is a huge variety and many different brands.

★ **RAMPAGE:** Rampage carries a great selection of clothing that is a bit more conservative and sophisticated, not to mention high quality. This store is reasonably priced and makes pieces that are better for nicer occasions.

★ **ROJAS:** To see the Rojas line of clothing (and their store) is to love it. It's not a matter of "Will I find something?"—it's a matter of "I want to own everything!" The fabric, styles, and designer, Freddie, are all fabulous!

★ **STEVE MADDEN:** Steve Madden is definitely one of my favorite shoe companies. All the shoes in the store are always great and come in a whole bunch of colors to choose from. Steve Madden shoes are also reasonably priced, which means every teen can have a couple of pairs of Steve Maddens in her closet without emptying her purse.

★ **TARGET:** I love Target for their great prices and designer looks! When I go to Target, I love to shop the little boy's clothing section: Usually, the larger sizes there will fit me and look great. I like that masculine/feminine look. Not to mention their inexpensive wife-beaters and thermals. I also like their accessory section, which includes jewelry, purses, and other miscellaneous stuff like leg warmers.

★ **TIFFANY & CO.:** Everyone knows Tiffany's has the most beautiful jewelry. I love their pieces because they are timeless and simply elegant.

★ **URBAN OUTFITTERS:** I love Urban Outfitters! They have a great selection of clothing from different brands like Triple 5 Soul and Diesel.

★ **VICTORIA'S SECRET:** My favorite bras and panties are from Victoria's Secret. I love everything, because it's so pretty and there are so many women there to help you choose a style of bra that will fit you best and give you the support you need. Plus, they are now carrying a great selection of active wear.

★ **VOOM:** Located in the Westside Pavilion in Los Angeles, this clothing line makes beautiful, unique pieces. Voom is a little more on the pricey side, but definitively worth the splurge.

★ **WAL-MART:** Everyone has heard about Wal-Mart, but I don't think many people regard it as one of their favorite stores. I really like Wal-Mart for their purses and little boy's clothing section.

★ **WET SEAL:** This clothing chain carries a variety of different lines. With more than 150 stores, it shouldn't be too hard to find one near you. Their prices are great!

★ **WINDSOR:** Windsor clothing chain has a great selection of clothing. In the back of all their stores they have a beautiful collection of fancy dresses that could be worn to a prom. The clothing in Windsor is normally in the neighborhood of $40 or more, depending on the article of clothing.

Yellow Pages

Here's a fast way to find my favorite stores and brands. I've listed the Web sites for companies that have them and phone numbers or e-mail addresses for those that don't.

ABERCROMBIE & FITCH
www.abercrombie.com

AKADEMIKS
www.akademiks.com

AMBER'S ESCAPADES
www.ambersescapades.com

AMERICAN EAGLE OUTFITTERS
www.ae.com

AMERICAN RAG
www.americanragcie.com

APPLE BOTTOMS
www.applebottoms.com

BABY PHAT
www.babyphat.com

BCBG
www.bcbg.com

BEBE
www.bebe.com

BELLA-CHIC TEASE
www.bella-chic.com

BEVERLY HILLS PIMPS & HO'S
www.beverlyhillspimpsandhos.com

BIJOU DRIVE
www.bijoudrive.com

BIZ
www.bizent.net

BLUE MARLIN
www.bluemarlincorp.com

BONGO
www.bongo.com

BONKNITS BY BONNIE
e-mail: bonniflowers@aol.com

CANDIES
www.candies.com

CATCH A FIRE
www.catchafireclothing.com

CHEYNE HAUK
e-mail: cheynehauk@yahoo.com

CHICA
www.chica1.com

CHINESE LAUNDRY
www.chineselaundry.com

CONVERSE
www.converse.com

CUSTO BARCELONA
www.custo-barcelona.com

DEMOSS JEANS
www.demossjeans.com

DIESEL
www.diesel.com

DOLLHOUSE
www.dollhouse.com

DORFMAN PACIFIC
www.dorfman-pacific.com

DOUGLAS FIR
323-651-5445

ECKO RED
www.eckored.com

ELAN
www.elan-usa.com

EOEO CLOTHING/ DEAR JOHN
e-mail: eoeoclothing@aol.com

FOOT LOCKER
www.footlocker.com

FOREVER 21 (XXI)
www.forever21.com

G UNIT
www.g-unitclothing.com

GANG RIO
www.gang-rio.com.br

GIRL STAR
www.girlstar.com

GORJANA
www.gorjana.com

GUESS
www.guess.com

HOT KISS
www.hotkiss.com

JAMES PERSE
www.jamesperse.com

JOHNNY GIRL
www.johnnyhandsome.net

JUICY COUTURE
www.juicycouture.com

JUNK FOOD FOREVER
www.junkfoodforever.com

LEATHEROCK
www.leatherock.com

LEE RIOT
www.leeriot.com

LITTLE EARTH
www.littlearth.com

LUCKY BRAND JEANS
www.luckybrandjeans.com

MACY'S
www.macys.com

MARCIANO
www.marciano.com

MARIANNA'S DESIGNER JEWELRY
www.mdj2.com

MECCA FEMME
www.meccafemme.com

MICA
e-mail: nisamica@aol.com
213-624-7611

MICHAEL ANTONIO
www.michaelantonio.com

MIGUEL TORRES
www.torres-miguel.com

MIKEN CLOTHING
www.mikenclothing.com

NEW YORK CITY SUBWAY LINE
www.nycsubwayline.com

NORDSTROM
www.nordstrom.com

OCEAN DRIVE CLOTHING
www.oceandriveclothing.com

ORIENT EXPRESS
e-mail: Jackiebshowroom@yahoo.com

PETER GRIMM HEADWEAR
www.petergrimm.com

PICASSO STYLE INC.
www.picassostyleinc.com

PLANET BODY
e-mail: planetbodyingrid@aol.com

RAMPAGE
www.rampage.com

ROACH KILLERS
(Designer: Alejandra Hernandez)
e-mail: Artbyme99@hotmail.com

ROCAWEAR
www.rocawear.com

ROJAS
e-mail: rojas@rojasonline.com

SAN FRANCISCO CITY LIGHTS
www.sfcitylights.com

SLEAZE
www.sleazehollywood.com

SPARKLICIOUS
e-mail: valeriejac@aol.com

STEVE MADDEN
www.stevemadden.com

SUPER LUCKY CAT
www.superluckycat.com

TARGET
www.target.com

TEAM DIVA
www.teamdiva.com

TIFFANY & CO.
www.tiffany.com

TIMBERLAND
www.timberland.com

TRIPLE 5 SOUL
www.triple5soul.com

URBAN OUTFITTERS
www.urbanoutfitters.com

VICTORIA'S SECRET
www.victoriassecret.com

VINTAGE PEANUTS
e-mail: randi.kagan@jemsportswear.com

VITIARE
e-mail: jackiebshowroom @yahoo.com

VOOM
e-mail: nisamica@aol.com

WAL-MART
www.walmart.com

WET SEAL
www.wetseal.com

WHITE BOY
www.whiteboy.com

WINDSOR
www.windsorclothing.com

XOXO
www.xoxo.com

YOUR SISTER'S MUSTACHE
www.ysmny.com

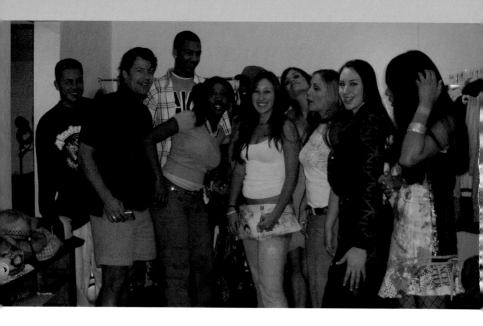

Special Thanks

I want to thank everyone who made this book possible. First, I would like to start with my mom, Linda. If it weren't for her guidance and push, I would never have dreamed of even writing a book. She was the one who suggested that I write my first, self-published book back in the 8th grade, when I swore to her that I wouldn't wear the same outfit twice throughout the entire year. She was responsible for submitting my book, *How to Be a Teen Fashionista*, to Fair Winds Press for consideration, as well as for getting in touch with the clothing companies. If it weren't for my mom, none of this would be happening. She believes in me with all her heart and is my biggest fan. I love you, Mom!

Secondly, I would like to thank my editor, Ellen Phillips. I was so lucky to work with someone who believed in me as much as my own family. I've gotten so used to our business correspondence through e-mails that now

that it's over, I miss it. Ellen really has spoiled me because I don't think there's a better editor out there.

I would like to give a very special thank you to the companies listed here. They trusted and believed in me. I thank them for their fabulous clothing, jewelry, shoes, and accessories. Their time, effort, and kindness will be forever appreciated. Without them, I could not have created the fashions in this book. In alphabetical order: Akademiks, Amber's Escapades, Beverly Hills Pimps & Ho's, Biz, Boom Boom Jeans, Catch A Fire, Cheyne Hauk, Chica, Converse, Custo, Ecko Red, EOEO/Dear John, Forever 21, G Unit, Gorjana, Hot Kiss, Johnny Girl, Junk Food Forever, Leatherock, Lee Riot, Little Earth, Lucky Brand Jeans, Marianna's Designer Jewelry, Mecca Femme, Mica, Michael Antonio, Miken, New York City Subway Line, Peter Grimm Headwear, Roach Killers, Rocawear,

Rojas, Sleaze, Steve Madden, Triple 5 Soul, Vintage Peanuts by Jem Sport, Voom, and Your Sister's Mustache.

I was fortunate to be grantd the use of the one-of-a-kind men's suits by Douglas Fir for this book. Thank you, Jon for taking a leap of faith with me when I walked into your store and asked to use your suits. Thank you Akademiks for providing me with all the clothing for my male models, and a special thanks to Simon Aaronson at Akademiks for all your time and efforts in helping make those outfits awesome!

Another special thank you goes to MAC Cosmetics for believing in me and this book. MAC contributed all the cosmetics used to make me and my models beautiful. Thank you so much, MAC!

There are a few people who I worked with personally from the companies I listed above. These people deserve recognition for their over-the-top efforts. In no special order, I would like to thank Shanda Standifer for your assistance above and beyond, Elissa Kravetz for always "stepping out" for me, Franco Nakagawa from Jackie B Showroom for going the extra mile, Meghan Bryan for making a girl's dream a reality, Hallie Tsabag for always being there when I need

her, Shelley Hancock for making us all beautiful, and Maria Harutunian for her friendship and inspiration.

It was once again a pleasure to work with Myk Mishoe, our location consultant. Myk is the creative genius behind the scenes. Thank you, Myk, for your insight, creativity, fabulous studio, and, last but not least, your friendship.

Another group of people I would like to thank are my female models (and good friends): Nikki Angel, Angie Llerena, Ashley Martinez, Carissa Micas, Jackie Szajer, and Aviona Williams. They worked so hard both days of the photo shoot. It's not as easy to be beautiful as it looks! I would also like to thank my male models: Todd Chisom, Tony Lunnon, Moses Obiarinze, Gavin Palmer, Edwin Rivas, Spencer Paysinger, and James Tomas.

Last, I want to thank a very special teacher at Beverly Hills High School, Mr. Albert. Mr. Albert duals as my woodshop teacher and coach for the wrestling team. I am his woodshop student and the manager of his wrestling team. Mr. Albert fully supported me during the ten weeks I wrote my book. He was patient and understanding, and he allowed me the freedom I needed to bring this book successfully to print. Thank you, Mr. Albert, for being the best teacher ever!

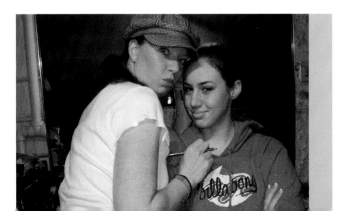

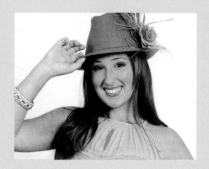

About the Author

Chase Koopersmith is 15 years old and lives in Beverly Hills with her mother, Linda, and two cats, Cookie and Rosie. Chase is currently a sophomore at Beverly Hills High School. In her free time, Chase can be found at any of the major shopping malls or bookstores in her area or shopping on Melrose. She also likes to hang out with friends, go to movies, listen to music, and read vampire novels.

Visit Chase on her Web site www.htbatf.com or www.howtobeateenfashionista.com for more great ideas.